On Equal Terms: Working with Disabled People

On Equal Terms: Working with Disabled People

Edited by

Sally French

BSc, MSc (Psych), MSc(Soc), GradDipPhys, DipTP
Lecturer, School of Health, Welfare and Community Education,
Open University, UK

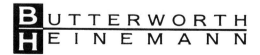

BUTTERWORTH
HEINEMANN

Butterworth-Heinemann Ltd
Linacre House, Jordan Hill, Oxford OX2 8DP

 A member of the Reed Elsevier plc group

OXFORD LONDON BOSTON
MUNICH NEW DELHI SINGAPORE SYDNEY
TOKYO TORONTO WELLINGTON

First published 1994

British Library Cataloguing in Publication Data
A catalogue record for this book is available from the British Library.

ISBN 0 7506 0751 3

Library of Congress Cataloguing in Publication Data
A catalogue record for this book is available from the Library of Congress.

Typeset by ROM Data Corporation Limited, Falmouth, Cornwall
Printed in Great Britain by Biddles Limited, Guildford and Kings Lynn

Contents

Contributors

Colin Barnes Cert Ed (FE), BA, PhD
Lecturer in Disability Studies, School of Sociology and Social Policy, University of Leeds. Research Director, British Council of Organizations of Disabled People (BCODP).

Ken Davis
Activist, author on disability issues and founder of many disability organizations.

Devala Dookun MCSP SRP
Senior Paediatric Physiotherapist, Child Development Centre, St George's Hospital, London.

Sally French BSc, MSc (Psych), MSc (Soc), GradDipPhys, DipTP
Lecturer, School of Health, Welfare and Community Education, Open University.

Chris Jones BA, DipCOT
Service Provision Manager, Society for the Welfare and Teaching of the Blind, Edinburgh and South-East Scotland. Formerly employed as Senior Occupational Therapist in the Learning Disabilities Directorate of North Mersey Community (NHS) Trust.

Paul Lawrence BEd, MPhil
Lecturer (Programme Co-ordinator), North Tyneside College of Further Education.

Jenny Morris BSc, PGCE, PhD
Freelance researcher, consultant, trainer and writer on disability issues.

Louise Silburn BA, IHSM
Performance Manager, Trent Regional Health Authority.

John Swain BSc, PGC, MSc, PhD
Senior Lecturer (Special Educational Needs), University of Northumbria.

Carole Thirlaway BA
Senior Teacher, Kiltonthorpe School, Cleveland.

Jan Walmsley BA, PGCE, MSc
Lecturer, School of Health, Welfare and Community Education, Open University.

Helen Westcott BSc
Research Officer, National Society for the Prevention of Cruelty to Children, London.

Preface

Over the last twenty years disabled people have become increasingly organized politically in a struggle to improve their situation. Disabled people are denied their basic rights of citizenship; they are segregated in 'special' institutions and denied access to education, employment, transport, information, housing and community facilities. Most disabled people live in poverty and are denied the services and equipment needed for a lifestyle of their choice. Even the most basic choices, such as when to get up and when to have a bath, are denied to many.

Disabled people have also been subject to the hostile and patronizing attitudes of non-disabled people, including health and welfare professionals and those who work for charities. They have been expected to play a particular role of passivity, gratitude, dependency and 'courage', and have sometimes become inwardly oppressed by internalizing these role expectations.

Although the assistance health professionals can offer disabled people is not denied, they can also be viewed as part of the problem. Health professionals work within the power structures which control disabled people's lives and maintain them in their disadvantaged state. Professional education has rarely addressed disability from a civil rights perspective, but rather has chosen to view it as the personal problem of individuals who happen to have impairments.

This situation of inequality, discrimination and prejudice is now being widely challenged by the growing disability movement.

The aim of this book is to explain the ideas and perspectives of the collective voice of disabled people and to offer suggestions on how the practice of nurses and therapists could be changed to enable them to work *with* disabled people as allies in their struggle. The book is concerned with the underlying social, psychological and political issues which affect the lives of disabled people regardless of their particular impairments. This having been said, it is fair to point out that the book is orientated towards physical and sensory impairment, although two chapters address learning difficulties specifically. Every effort has been made to ensure that the book is accessible to those readers with no background knowledge in this area. It is extensively referenced to assist those readers who require further information.

I would like to thank all those who have helped, and continue to help, me develop my understanding of disability. These include Vic Finkelstein, Mike Oliver, Jenny Morris, Lois Keith, David Hevey, Colin Barnes and Ken Davis. Thanks are also extended to Caroline Makepeace and Tim Brown of Butterworth–Heinemann for their constant encouragement, faith and good humour, and to all the authors who have contributed chapters to this book.

I am grateful to The Open University for allowing me to re-print Jenny Morris's chapter 'Prejudice' from the following publication:

Swain, J., Finkelstein, V., French, S. and Oliver, M. (eds) (1993) *Disabling Barriers—Enabling Environments*, Sage, London

I am grateful to the following publishers for allowing existing work to be used or modified for use in this book:

Taylor and Francis for allowing me to use the following article as the basis for chapter 10 'Researching disability':

French, S. (1992) Researching disability: the way forward. *Disability and Rehabilitation*, **14 (4)**, 183–186

Jill Whitehouse of The Chartered Society of Physiotherapy for allowing me to use the following article as the basis for chapter 13 'Disabled people from minority ethnic groups':

French, S. (1992) Health care in a multi-ethnic society. *Physiotherapy*, **78 (3)**, 174–180

Blackwell Publishers for allowing me to use the following article as the basis for chapter 16 'Disabled health professionals':

French, S. (1988) Experiences of disabled health and caring professionals. *Sociology of Health and Illness*, **10 (2)**, 170–188

I am grateful The Open University and Louise Silburn for allowing me to abridge the following chapter for use in chapter 18 'Innovative practice':

Silburn, L. (1993) A social model in a medical world: the development of the integrated living team as part of the strategy for younger disabled people in North Derbyshire. In *Disabling Barriers—Enabling Environments*, (eds J. Swain, V. Finkelstein, S. French and M. Oliver), Sage, London

Finally I would like to thank the many physiotherapy and nursing students I have taught over the years who have enabled me to gain the necessary expertise and confidence to write this book.

Sally French

1

What is disability?

Sally French

There is no simple way of defining disability, it can be viewed from many perspectives. Within every society there are competing models of disability with some being more dominant than others at different times. These models, or abstract representations, although often in conflict, gradually influence and modify each other. The models put forward by powerful groups within society, such as the medical profession and the government, tend to dominate the models of less powerful groups, such as disabled people themselves.

It is very important to explore the ways in which disability is defined, as well as who defines it, for attitudes and behaviour towards disabled people, professional practice and the running of institutions, such as rehabilitation centres and hospitals, are based, at least in part, on these definitions. As Oliver points out, 'the "lack of fit" between able-bodied and disabled people's definitions is more than just a semantic quibble for it has important implications both for the provision of services and the ability to control one's life' (1993a: 61).

The individualistic model of disability

Most models of disability are based upon the assumption that the problems and difficulties disabled people experience are a direct result of their individual physical, sensory or intellectual impairments. This position is articulated most clearly in the medical model of disability.

The medical model of disability

The medical and health and welfare professions are dominant and powerful agents in defining disability. The medical model of disability has led people to view it in terms of disease process, abnormality and personal tragedy. Brechin and Liddiard (1981) point out that the medical model has guided and dominated clinical practice with the resulting assumption that both problems and solutions lie within disabled people rather than within society. The medical approach has been insufficiently broad to concern itself with disability from the disabled person's point of view, or the disabling effects of society itself. Oliver states, 'this medical approach produces definitions of disability which are partial and limited and which fail to take into account wider aspects of disability' (1990: 5).

Because the medical model lies at the heart of clinical practice it may be difficult for health and welfare professionals to consider changing their attitudes and behaviour towards disability and disabled people. McKnight (1981) points out that the existence of many professional roles are dependent on viewing disability in terms of the medical model, and that the very tools and techniques which professionals have at their disposal serve to define and individualize problems. Oliver (1993b) is of the opinion that the medical model of disability may serve the needs of professionals more than the needs of disabled people and Ryan and Thomas, talking of people with learning difficulties, state:

> Medical model thinking tends to support the status quo. The subnormality of the individual rather than the subnormality of the environment, tends to be blamed for any inadequacies. . . . Within most institutions staff have a vested interest in not questioning the quality of the patients' environment too radically, for they themselves are part of that environment. (1987: 27)

Thomas and Ryan also believe that although the causes of learning difficulties, if known at all, are usually related to socio-economic conditions such as malnutrition and poverty, medicine has concerned itself mainly with the study of rare syndromes, and its emphasis on abnormality and incurability has justified the appalling conditions under which people with learning difficulties have had to live. They believe that learning difficulties provide a case study of the medicalization of a social problem.

Individualizing disability is certainly not a practice peculiar to medicine, though other professions and institutions have undoubtedly been influenced by the medical model. Shearer (1981), for example, notes that the first official aim of the International Year of Disabled People in 1981 was, 'helping disabled people in their physical and psychological adjustment to society'.

Individualistic professional definitions, those from both inside and outside the health and welfare professions, certainly have the potential to do serious harm. The medicalization of learning difficulties, which is now being questioned, is one example. Another is oralism, the belief that deaf people should dispense with sign language and learn to rely exclusively on lip reading. The philosophy and practice of oralism has led Ladd (1990) to believe that human beings are capable of disabling each other far more profoundly than could any impairment. It is certainly most unlikely that a deaf person would ever have devised such a plan. (For further information about oralism and the backlash against it, the reader is referred to Ladd (1988) and Gregory and Hartley (1991)).

Other institutions within society also take a medicalized, individualistic stance to disability. This was so until recently in education where children were categorized fairly rigidly in terms of their impairments. It eventually became apparent that categorizing children in this way, while paying scant attention to their other characteristics and attributes, made little sense, and in the 1981 Education Act the broader notion of 'special educational needs' emerged, as well as a resolve to educate disabled children in mainstream schools.

The concept of 'special educational needs' has itself been criticized for focusing on individual children, rather than on educational policy and practice. The criteria and assessment procedures for extra help or support are heavily based on tests of impairment. Oliver states, 'The individual model sees the problems that disabled people experience as being a direct consequence of their disability. The major task of the professional is therefore to adjust the individual to the particular disabling condition' (1983: 15). Ellis (1993) found that professionals, when assessing disabled people, believed that need arose directly from impairment, and that professional interventions were aimed at enabling the disabled individual to cope safely and independently.

By individualizing disability the effect of the environment upon the lives of disabled people is not addressed. Indeed the environments imposed upon disabled people in the name of treatment, for example mental handicap hospitals and Young Disabled Units, can have detrimental effects leading to greater dependency and an increase in existing problems of function or behaviour. In addition, as Mittler (1979) points out, people subjected to such environments may be the very people who are most susceptible to their adverse effects.

Blaxter (1976) notes that definitions of disability have become wider and more complex with disagreement, in many instances, over whether the problems of disablement should be the concern of the medical profession at all. Despite this, and the expansion of other professional groups and institutions, the medical profession has considerable control over non-medical decisions such as housing, employment and education. This has led some disabled people to complain that although their particular impairments give rise to no medical problems and cannot be improved by medical intervention, medicine has nonetheless had a dominant influence over important decisions affecting their lives (French, 1987). Finkelstein (1991a) is of the opinion that issues relating to disability would be better placed in the Department of the Environment, rather than the Department of Health, and that important new disciplines in engineering and architecture need to be developed.

It should never be assumed that there is consensus regarding the definitions of disability or illness between or within the medical and welfare professions. Mental illness, for example, is viewed in physiological, psychological and sociological terms (Tyrer and Steinberg, 1987; French, 1989) and even as a myth (Szasz, 1961). Similarly one physiotherapist may define disability very differently from another, or regard people with different impairments in diverse ways. Nurses and occupational therapists may not agree on their definitions, nor speech and language therapists with doctors. Our perceptions of disability are shaped by a multitude of factors not least of which is professional education, socialization and specialization. The effect of this is often to produce a narrowed perception of disability which can easily give rise to conflict or ineffective communication with both disabled people and colleagues.

Administrative models of disability

Administrative models of disability tend to be rigid and dichotomous and are often written into legislation and acts of parliament with legal implications. These models usually relate to specific areas of life such as education and employment, and are used to assess whether or not people are eligible for certain benefits or compensation. The definitions of disability which arise from these models, as well as the measurements and criteria used for assessment, almost always relate to people's impairments rather than the physical and social environments in which they are obliged to live. One of the problems with rigid definitions such as these is that, owing to the complexity of disability, disabled people rarely fit into the neat boxes administrators provide. For this reason administrative definitions are often viewed as unfair and divisive. It is not uncommon for severely disabled people to be denied benefits because their impairments or disabilities do not fit the rigid criteria demanded. It was not until 1990, for example, that people who are both deaf and blind were eligible for the mobility allowance.

Rigid definitions of disability can be harmful in other ways. As noted above, until recent times children with a given impairment, such as blindness or partial hearing, were educated in special schools regardless of their other characteristics and attributes, the decision being based largely on tests of impairment. Similarly, until 1971 children whose IQ scores fell below a certain level were said to be 'ineducable', but it is now known that an individual's IQ score is a less than perfect predictor of ability and social capacity, and that children with learning difficulties need more, rather than less, education.

This having been said, loose administrative definitions can be even more dangerous than rigid ones because large numbers of people can be readily labelled 'disabled' and treated accordingly. Under the Mental Deficiency Acts of 1913 and 1927, for example, people could be categorized as 'mentally deficient' without any reference to their personal circumstances or intellect, and many were detained merely because of socially disapproved behaviour, such as becoming pregnant, having emotional problems, or failing to give the right answers to a series of questions (Laing and McQuarrie, 1989; Potts and Fido, 1991; Humphries and Gordon, 1992).

Health and welfare professionals are forced to work within the framework of administrative definitions, yet such is their power that the rules can often be bent. For example, it is not unusual for visually-impaired people to be refused entry to the blind person's register by one consultant ophthalmologist, but be placed on it with little ado by another. There are various advantages to being registered 'blind' rather than 'partially sighted' but the tests adopted are crude and the dividing line between the two categories is ill-defined. Thus the decisions made depend, at least in part, on the doctor's and the disabled person's attitudes towards blindness and their ability and willingness to negotiate with each other.

Finkelstein (1991a) uses the term 'administrative model' in a rather different way. He views it as an overarching model which encompasses those models of disability where disabled people are thought to be in need of care and ministration by others; he refers to it as the 'cure or care' approach. For Finkelstein the medical model is merely a variant of the administrative model; thus if the medical profession were to lose its power the work of ministering to disabled people would be taken over by some other agency. This is happening, to some extent, as a result of 'care in the community' policies.

The philanthropic model of disability

Charities have tended to portray disabled people as helpless, sad, courageous and in need of care and protection (Scott-Parker, 1989; Barnes, 1992). Such images, presumably believed to be the most effective means of raising money, are now thought to have caused considerable harm to disabled people by perpetuating damaging stereotypes and misconceptions. Charities frequently mislead the public in the type of client they portray. Organizations for visually impaired people, for example, have tended to depict a disproportionate number of blind children with no additional impairments, whereas in reality the majority of their clients are elderly, partially sighted, or multiply disabled: people who are, perhaps, less likely to arouse emotion, public sympathy and support.

Many disabled people find images presented by charities offensive, as their demonstrations against 'telethons' illustrate. Disabled people have complained that these and similar events serve to give publicity to companies and to provide entertainment for non-disabled people, as well as boosting their egos as they publicly donate large sums of money (*Disability Now*, 1990). Organizations such as the Campaign to Stop Patronage and the British Council of Organization of Disabled People, believe the funds given to charities would be far better used by disabled people directly to campaign politically for their rights.

In recent years the portrayal of disabled people has, however, become a little more positive. The front cover of the magazine *CONTACT* (1990), published by The Royal Association for Disability and Rehabilitation (RADAR), for example, shows a severely disabled boy using a computer, and the magazine of the Down's Syndrome Association (1989), is full of positive images including notice of a forthcoming wedding and successful stories of educational integration. Images such as these, however, can be just as misleading and damaging as negative ones, for they tend to concentrate on exceptional disabled people, thereby denying or minimizing the considerable problems that the majority face. They underline the message that society expects disabled people to overcome what are viewed as *their* problems, to be 'normal' or even superhuman. (For further information on the ways in which charities portray disabled people, the reader is referred to chapter 3.)

Lay models of disability

Lay models of disability are diverse and constantly changing; they are influenced by other models such as those presented by charities and the medical profession. Models from the past, from religion and from other cultures, such as the association between disability and sin, and disability and virtue, may still linger and are sometimes reinforced in novels and plays (Karph, 1986; Barnes, 1992). Negative images of disabled people depicting them as sad, pathetic and dangerous, are also frequently represented in the arts of today.

Most people have a rather simplistic and superficial understanding of disability. For example, McConkey and McCormack (1983), reporting on various surveys conducted among people in Ireland, found that over half mentioned wheelchairs when asked 'What type of people do you think of when you think of the disabled or the handicapped?'. A further 25 per cent mentioned a physical impairment, with less than half understanding the difference between 'mentally ill' and 'mentally handicapped'. A poll conducted for MENCAP in 1982 gave similar findings. Taking all these polls together over 20 per cent of those surveyed defined disability in terms of 'people who cannot do things for themselves'.

Disability of a family member will be defined according to the interests and beliefs of that person and his or her family, which in turn will be influenced by prevailing cultural beliefs, attitudes and practices. A child with a physical impairment may be considered very disabled in a family whose main interest is sport, but hardly disabled at all in a family with more sedentary interests. Likewise a child who finds difficulty reading may be seen as very disabled in a highly intellectual family but not in a family with little interest in academic success. What is and what is not regarded as a disability is also reflected in social structures and values. Learning difficulties, for example, have become more disabling over the course of this century as the ability to read and cope with complex situations has become more important. Humphries and Gordon (1992) in their book about disability in the first half of the twentieth century, showed how, for many families, disability was a taboo subject causing shame and disappointment. These feelings were often internalized by disabled children who could not talk about their disabilities within the family.

Shakespeare (1975) points out that age can influence how disability is viewed by both the disabled person and others. Impairment or illness may be considered 'normal' or less tragic in old age depending on the particular family and culture. Disability in girls may be accepted and tolerated more readily than disability in boys, because the traditional role of the female has tended towards greater dependency. Thus ideas and perceptions of disability cannot be divorced from wider attitudes and beliefs about age and gender.

Self-definitions of disability

The social model

In the past it has been considered unnecessary to discover how disabled people view their situation. Like most under-privileged minority groups their views have been disregarded and suppressed. Disabled people have traditionally been considered dependent and in need of care. This attitude has led to the models of non-disabled people being thrust upon them. With the growing disability movement this situation has started to change. Oliver states:

> From the 1950s onwards . . . there was a growing realisation that if particular social problems were to be resolved or at least ameliorated, then nothing more or less than a fundamental redefinition of the problem was necessary. (1990: 3)

Although it should be borne in mind that disabled people form a heterogeneous group, with widely differing attitudes, there is growing evidence that their views of disability are thoroughly out of tune with those of professional workers. Oliver (1990) believes that whereas professionals view disability as stemming from the functional limitations of impaired individuals, disabled people believe that they stem from the failure of the social and physical environment to take account of their needs. Safilios-Rothschild (1976) points out that alternative solutions and innovative plans presented by disabled people have often been regarded as unrealistic by professional 'experts' who tend to view disabled people within the confines of a stereotyped role.

The following definitions of disability are based upon those of the former organization The Physically Impaired Against Segregation (UPIAS) (1976) and Disabled People's International (an international umbrella group of disabled people):

Impairment

Impairment is the lack of part or all of a limb, or having a defective limb, organ or mechanism of the body.

Disability

> Disability is the loss or limitation of opportunities that prevents people who have impairments from taking part in the normal life of the community on an equal level with others due to physical and social barriers. (Finkelstein and French, 1993: 28)

These and similar definitions have been adopted by politically active organizations of disabled people. They will be used to define impairment and disability throughout this book.

Oliver (1990) regards disabled people's views as constituting a social model of disability, where the problems are seen not within the individual disabled person but within society. Thus the person who uses a wheelchair is not disabled by paraplegia but by building design, lack of lifts, rigid work practices and the attitudes of others.

Similarly the visually-impaired person is not disabled by lack of sight, but by lack of Braille, cluttered pavements and stereotypical ideas about blindness. Finkelstein (1981) has argued that non-disabled people would be equally disabled if the environment was not designed with their needs in mind. Oliver (1990) contends that as the debate has occurred against a backdrop of discrimination and the struggle of disabled people against it, the neutral term 'social model' could just as well be replaced by the more politically laden term 'social oppression model'. It is important to remember that impairment itself is frequently socially produced, for example by malnourishment, poverty and war.

In recent years a number of disabled people, particularly women, have sought to extend the social model of disability to include impairment. Crow (1992) and French (1993) believe that it has been necessary for disabled people to provide a clear, unambiguous definition of disability to bring about political change. Admitting that there may be a negative side to disability, or highlighting problems which cannot be readily solved by social or environmental manipulation, may undermine the campaign. This has led to disabled activists ignoring impairment which has become something of a taboo word. Yet as Crow points out 'an impairment such as pain or chronic illness may curtail an individual's activities so much that the restriction of the outside world becomes irrelevant' (1992: 9). She points out that disability is not always insignificant or positive and believes that when disabled people ignore impairment they do so at considerable cost to themselves. Shakespeare agrees; he states 'It is important not to ignore differences between impairments, despite the tendency of writers to gloss over difference in favour of the totalizing and unifying role of oppression' (1993: 255).

These criticisms of the social model in no way invalidate it. Most of the disabled critics are merely aiming to increase its usefulness and power. As Crow explains:

> Integrating all the external and internal factors into the social model is vital if we are to understand fully the disability–impairment equation. This does not in any way undermine the social model, nor should it weaken our resolve for change. . . . Disability is still socially created, still unacceptable, and still there to be changed, but integrating impairment into the equation gives us the best route to creating a world that includes us all. (1992: 9)

Who are disabled people?

At the level of impairment there is a problem deciding who is and who is not disabled. Does a mild stammer constitute a speech disorder, and should a person with a limp be regarded as physically disabled? People are frequently said to be 'disabled' when they fall outside an accepted norm of function or behaviour, thus the concept of disability ultimately rests upon a social judgement.

Ladd (1988) explains that many profoundly-deaf people do not adhere to the notion that they are disabled, but rather prefer to view themselves as a linguistic and cultural minority, one which was very nearly annihilated by the suppression of sign language and the practice of oralism. Finkelstein has challenged this view, however. He states:

> It seems that when people with a hearing impairment identify themselves as language oppressed but not disabled, while at the same time they see people with a mobility impairment as disabled (but not as mobility oppressed) they are attributing medical labels to others in exactly the same way they reject such labels for themselves. (1991b: 269)

If disability is defined in terms of the social model, it becomes easier to comprehend who is and who is not disabled. Stevens defines a disabled person as 'someone who as a consequence of their impairment experiences social oppression of whatever kind' and disablism as 'a form of social oppression towards disabled people' (1992: 16). Thus disability results from an interaction between impairment and the physical and social world.

Systems of classification

The International Classification of Disease (ICD)

The International Classification of Disease (ICD) classifies disease in terms of its aetiology, pathology and manifestations, but does not consider the effects of these on the individual; it is a classification system based entirely upon the medical model of disease. The system works reasonably well when considering acute illness, such as pneumonia, but is unsatisfactory when attempting to describe or understand chronic illness or disability. For this reason a new and broader system was accepted by the World Health Organization in 1980.

The International Classification of Impairments, Disabilities and Handicaps (ICIDH)

This classification system takes a broader view of disease and impairment than the ICD by considering the consequences of it from the affected individual's point of view. The increase in chronic, long-term disease and the decrease in acute disease has made the ICD less and less useful. The ICIDH also attempts to classify and describe the consequences of impairments, such as absence of an eye or a limb, which cannot be described in terms of disease. 'Impairment', 'disability' and 'handicap' are defined as follows:

Impairment

Any loss or abnormality of psychological, physiological or anatomical structure or function. Thus an impairment could range from a scar on the skin to the malfunction of the liver or the heart.

Disability

Any restriction or lack of ability to perform an activity, as a result of impairment, in a manner or within the range considered normal for a human being, for example the ability to climb the stairs or walk to the shops.

Handicap

A disadvantage for a given individual, resulting from an impairment or a disability, that limits or prevents the fulfilment of a role for that individual (depending on such factors as age, sex and social and cultural factors). Handicap refers to the disadvantage the individual encounters, as a result of the impairment and/or the disability, when compared with his or her peers.

This scheme illustrates that the concepts of 'impairment', 'disability' and 'handicap' are independent of each other, though they can also co-exist. Take, for example, a person with a facial deformity or skin disease which, using this system, would be classed as an impairment. People with an impairment such as this will probably experience no disability, as independent living is unlikely to be impeded. Nevertheless, they may experience considerable handicap, being denied employment in certain occupations, or full social integration. A person with a facial deformity or a skin disorder may very well experience more handicap than someone with a substantial disability, and a person with a mild disability may experience more handicap than a person with a severe disability.

Thomas is of the opinion that handicap is the result of an interaction between impairment, disability, the psychological attributes of the individual, the available resources and prevailing social attitudes. He believes that the concept of 'handicap' is a value judgement and states 'to move from impairment to handicap is to cover the distance from symptoms to social role' (1982: 7).

The concepts of 'illness' and 'disease' are also independent of 'impairment', 'disability' and 'handicap'. For example, a person with rheumatoid arthritis has a disease, may well feel ill and is also likely to be disabled. On the other hand, someone who loses a limb as a result of an accident, or is partially sighted as a result of albinism, can hardly be described as ill or diseased such people may, in fact, be extremely fit and healthy. It is unfortunate that disability is so often automatically equated with disease and illness. Harrison (1987) complains that the term 'chronically sick' is often used synonymously with disability even though those with the most profound disabilities can be quite free of disease. Oliver (1983b) believes that the Chronically Sick and Disabled Person's Act encourages these connections which are often erroneous.

The ICIDH has come under severe criticism by organizations controlled by disabled people, and has been rejected by the international organization Disabled People's International (IDP). Although the system moves away from a narrow medical definition and acknowledges that disability has social dimensions, both disability and handicap are viewed as *arising* from impairment rather than from social and environmental causes, and the social and physical environment are taken for granted and assumed to be fixed.

The system fails to address issues of central importance to disabled people, such as their education, employment and housing, and the concept of 'normality' is accepted uncritically with little recognition of its cultural and temporal determinants.

Conclusion

Disabled people's definitions of the problems they encounter, and the appropriate solutions to them, are generally given insufficient weight in the education and practice of professional health and welfare workers. This situation has given rise to countless examples of inappropriate, oppressive and damaging practices and policies.

Disabled people define their situation not in terms of individual impairment but in terms of social oppression. By doing so they are not implying that medical intervention is wrong, or that it cannot be sensible, helpful or vital. What disabled people are demanding of professional workers is a broadening of their perspective on disability and a relinquishing of their power.

References

Barnes, C. (1992) *Disabling Imagery and the Media*, The British Council of Organizations of Disabled People and Ryburn Publishing Limited, Halifax

Blaxter, M. (1976) *The Meaning of Disability*, Heinemann, London

Brechin, A. and Liddiard, P. (1981) *Look at it This Way—New Perspectives in Rehabilitation*, Hodder & Stoughton, Sevenoaks

CONTACT (1990) Journal of the Royal Association for Disability and Rehabilitation, Summer, **64**

Crow, L. (1992) Renewing the social model of disability. *Coalition*, July, Greater Manchester Coalition of Disabled People, 5–9

Disability Now, Telethon is a modern day freak show (1990), 3 July

Down's Syndrome Association News (1989) Spring

Ellis, K. (1993) *Squaring the Circle. User and Carer Participation in Needs Assessment*, Joseph Rowntree Foundation, London

Finkelstein, V. (1981) To deny or not to deny disability. In *Handicap in a Social World*, (eds A. Brechin, P. Liddiard and J. Swain), Hodder & Stoughton, Sevenoaks

Finkelstein, V. (1991a) Disability: an administrative challenge. In Oliver M. (ed.) *Social Work, Disabled People and Disabling Environments*, Jessica Kingsley, London

Finkelstein, V. (1991b) 'We' are not disabled, 'you' are. In *Constructing Deafness*, (eds S. Gregory and C. M. Hartley), Pinter Publishers, London

Finkelstein, V. and French, S. (1993) Towards a psychology of disability. In *Disabling Barriers—Enabling Environments*, (eds J. Swain, V. Finkelstein, S. French and M. Oliver), Sage, London

French, S. (1987) The medicine epidemic. *Therapy Weekly*, **11 (34)** 4

French, S. (1989) Models of mental illness. *Therapy Weekly*, **16 (1)** 7

French, S. (1993) Disability, impairment or something in between? In *Disabling Barriers—Enabling Environments*, (eds Swain J, Finkelstein V., French S. and Oliver M.) Sage, London

Gregory, S. and Hartley, G. M. (1991) (eds) *Constructing Deafness*, Pinter Publishers, London

Harrison, J. (1987) *Severe Physical Disability*, Cassell, London

Humphries, S. and Gordon, P. (1992) *Out of Sight: the Experience of Disability 1900–1950*, Northcote House, Plymouth

International Classification of Impairments, Disabilities and Handicaps (1980) World Health Organization

Karph, A. (1986) *Doctoring the Media*, Routledge, London

Ladd, P. (1988) The modern deaf community. In *British Sign Language*, (D. Miles), BBC Books, London

Ladd, P. (1990) Language oppression and hearing impairment. In the book of readings of the disability equality pack *Disability—Changing Practice* (K665x), Open University, Milton Keynes

Laing, J. and McQuarrie, D. (1989) *50 Years in the System*, Mainstream Publishing Company, Edinburgh

McConkey, R. and McCormack, B. (1983) *Breaking Barriers: Educating People about Disability*, Souvenir Press, London

McKnight, J. (1981) Professionalised service and disabling help. In *Handicap in a Social World*, (eds A. Brechin, P. Liddiard and J. Swain), Hodder & Stoughton, Sevenoaks

Mittler, P. (1979) *People Not Patients: Problems and Policies in Mental Handicap*, Methuen, London

Oliver, M. (1983) *Social Work and Disabled People*, Macmillan, London

Oliver, M. (1990) *The Politics of Disablement*, Macmillan, London

Oliver, M. (1993a) Disability, citizenship and empowerment. Workbook 2 of the course *The Disabling Society* (K665), Open University, Milton Keynes

Oliver, M. (1993b) Disability and dependency: a creation of industrial societies? In *Disabling Barriers—Enabling Environments*, (eds J. Swain, V. Finkelstein, S. French and M. Oliver), Sage, London

Potts, M. and Fido, R. (1991) *'A Fit Person to be Removed': Personal Accounts of Life in a Mental Deficiency Institution*, Northcote House, Plymouth

Ryan, J. and Thomas, F. (1987) *The Politics of Mental Handicap*, Free Association Books, London

Safilios-Rothschild, C. (1976) Disabled person's self-definitions and their implications for rehabilitation. In *Rehabilitation: Supplementary Readings*, (V. Finkelstein), Open University Press, Milton Keynes

Scott-Parker, S. (1989) *They Aren't in the Brief*, King's Fund Centre, London

Shakespeare, R. (1975) *The Psychology of Handicap*, Methuen, London

Shakespeare, T. (1993) Disabled people's self-organisation: a new social movement? *Disability, Handicap and Society*, **8 (3)**, 249–264

Shearer, A. (1981) *Disability: Whose Handicap?*, Basil Blackwell, Oxford

Stevens, A. (1992) *Disability Issues: Developing Anti-discriminatory Practice*, Central Council for Education and Training in Social Work, London

Szasz, T. S. (1961) *The Myth of Mental Illness*, Harper & Row, New York

Thomas, D. (1982) *The Experience of Handicap*, Methuen, London

Tyrer, P. and Steinberg, D. (1987) *Models for Mental Disorder*, John Wiley, Chichester

UPIAS (1976) *Fundamental Principles of Disability*, Union of the Physically Impaired Against Segregation, London

2

Dimensions of disability and impairment

Sally French

The ways in which people experience disability and impairment depend on many interacting factors including social status, personality, personal history and environment. It was noted in chapter 1, for example, that a flight of steps can create disability and that the effects of an impairment vary with the person's interests and employment. In this chapter the following four factors, considered to be central to the experience of disability, will be discussed:

1. The point in life at which the impairment is acquired.
2. The visibility of the impairment.
3. The comprehensibility of the impairment and disability to others.
4. The presence or absence of illness.

Many of the psychological and social aspects of disability can be understood by analysing these and other factors. It is important to realize, however, that generalizations regarding impairment and disability merely provide ideas and possible explanations, never 'the truth' about any particular person.

The point in life at which the impairment is acquired

Impairment can arise at any time of life. The psychological and social effects of impairment and the disability which may accompany it are likely to differ according to the time of life at which it occurred.

If an impairment is present at birth or arises in early childhood many areas of development are at risk of disruption or delay, even those not directly associated with the impairment. Take, for example, children with cerebral palsy who are restricted in their ability to move around freely. Shakespeare (1975) believes that this situation has the potential to affect their cognitive development adversely, as they are less able to learn through exploration. Perceptual development, such as the appreciation and understanding of spatial relationships, may also be affected, as its full development is partly determined by movement and active manipulation of the environment.

Emotional, language and social development might also show delay in children with motor impairments; they may be dependent on adults far longer than usual, and their restricted mobility may mean that fewer demands are placed upon them. Their needs may be anticipated so readily that language is delayed and opportunities to play with other children may be limited or lacking (Lewis, 1987). Thus an impairment of the motor system threatens to disrupt many areas of development.

Whatever the impairment, a similar pattern holds. In the case of visual impairment a very important channel for learning is lost, this may be exacerbated by difficulty in moving safely and lack of incentive to move in the absence of visual stimuli. Lewis (1987) notes that visually impaired children are delayed in many aspects of their motor development including reaching forward, rolling and pushing up to sitting, as well as standing and walking independently. This lack of movement, as well as fear on the part of others that the child will come to harm, may disrupt social interaction and retard social development. The visually-impaired child may be given insufficient opportunities to take responsibility and to make mistakes, with a subsequent delay in emotional development.

The visually impaired child's language development may also be delayed. Burlington (1979) found that the vocabulary of visually impaired children develops more slowly than that of sighted children. The visually impaired child may have less experience of the world than other children and less to talk about. Lewis (1987) notes that visually impaired children have a qualitatively different experience of the environment than other people, including their parents and immediate carers. This may inhibit the acquisition of language as it is often heavily based on what we see, particularly when we interact with young children.

The notion that blind people have superior touch and hearing appears to be a misconception. Lewis states that 'there is no evidence to support the claim that the sensory apparatus of the blind child is actually more acute; she just uses the senses she has more effectively' (1987: 38). Lewis goes on to explain that blind children do less well than sighted children on a wide range of tactile and auditory tasks, although the differences lessen and disappear as the children get older. Sighted children, when blind-folded, tend to cope better than blind children on these tasks. Lewis suggests that this is because sight helps us to integrate information from all of our senses and to understand our other experiences; thus lack of sight clearly has the potential to delay the cognitive development of visually impaired children.

Murphy and O'Driscoll (1989) make a strong case for the involvement of physiotherapists in the lives of young visually-impaired children and their carers.

One advantage of congenital impairment is that the brains of young children are physiologically and anatomically malleable and will tend to develop in such a way as to maximize function. Thus a young child who injures the area of the brain responsible for language has the potential to regain this skill. This process is less successful when the brain is more mature. Similarly, the visual centre of the brain of a baby born with defective eyes is likely to develop in such a way as to maximize vision. This would not be possible if the same eye condition were acquired later in life. This is why it is so important that children be given the opportunity and encouraged to function within their area of impairment, provided it does not inhibit more satisfactory means of function and exploration, for example by the use of a wheelchair, or become a burden to them or their families. It also explains why a temporary period of loss, for example of sight or hearing, can be so detrimental, for it may occur at a particularly critical stage in the development of the brain.

Walker and Crawley (1983) state that the development of disabled children can be normal, absent, delayed, abnormal or compensatory. In the last case children may find an unusual way of achieving their goals, for example using their feet to manipulate objects rather than their hands, or using audible signals, which most people ignore, to compensate for lack of sight. Examples of abnormal development, according to Crawley, are rocking backwards and forwards, which is sometimes seen in blind children, and self-injurious behaviour, sometimes witnessed in children with learning difficulties. These behaviours can often be explained in terms of an interaction between the impairment and the environment; blind children may rock because they are under-stimulated, and the self-injurious behaviour of children with learning difficulties may be a symptom of frustration or boredom. Many disabled children have been subjected to impoverished institutional environments which in themselves can give rise to many adverse secondary effects and can be far more disruptive to human development than impairment (Oswin, 1978; Shearer, 1980). The disabling social and physical structures within society, such as lack of access to buildings, continue to impoverish the lives of many disabled people.

The areas of development which can be disrupted or delayed in children with motor and visual impairments are summarized in Figure 2.1.

This sequence of events is not inevitable but rather depends upon the limitations imposed by the impairment, parental and social attitudes and behaviour, the individual characteristics of the child,

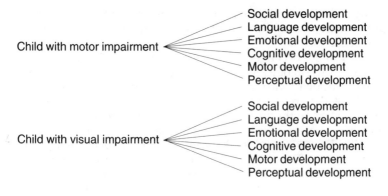

Figure 2.1

available resources and the social and physical environment in which the child and his or her family are placed. The situation will, of course, be complicated if the child has multiple impairments (see Brudenell, 1986).

As well as the threat of disruption to all areas of development which an impairment imposes, disabled children are likely to be socialized into a particular role during their formative years. This may have an adverse effect on their confidence and self-esteem.

An important aspect of the health professional's role is to minimize or prevent developmental delay by informing parents or carers of the potential problems and working with them to devise developmental programmes specific to each child. The parents or carers of a visually-impaired child, for example, may be helped to participate, at least in part, in the child's experience of touch and sound and to base activities around these senses. The parents or carers of a motor-impaired child can be helped to maximize stimulation and to encourage interaction. Families must be consulted when devising interventions to ensure that their ideas are included and that all activities fit in with family routines and do not become unduly stressful, time-consuming, or boring for any family member. Lewis (1987) provides detailed information of the development of children with a wide range of impairments, as well as interventions which may be used to enhance development and minimize detrimental effects. (For further information on the families of disabled people, the reader is referred to chapter 12).

People who acquire an impairment in later childhood or adult life have the advantage that they have been non-disabled until that point in time. For example, when people become deaf in adulthood they will usually have acquired language and the ability to read and write fluently. Similarly those who lose their sight in later life will have full knowledge of the visual world on which to draw; their mobility and orientation will, in fact, frequently surpass that of congenitally blind people, although skills such as braille reading tend to be more difficult to acquire. Lewis (1987) notes that the experience of sight may help people to use their other senses more effectively.

People who become disabled in old age, by far the majority, may find their situation particularly difficult owing to the fact that they frequently have multiple impairments. Thus the older person who starts to go deaf may also have a visual impairment, and the person who becomes paralysed following a stroke may already have arthritis or a heart complaint. The older person who becomes paraplegic may simply lack sufficient physical strength to manage as a younger person might. It is important, however, not to be ageist (French, 1992a), many older people cope with impairment and disability as effectively as younger people.

Although childhood is the period in life of most rapid development, it should not be forgotten that people continue to develop throughout their lives. Those who acquire an impairment in adulthood, therefore, may find their social, sexual, emotional and cognitive opportunities and development restricted. They may also experience prejudice, discrimination and hostile reactions. A person with ataxia following a head injury, for example, may fail to find employment or to integrate fully in society because of the attitudes and behaviour of others as well as an inaccessible environment. This may lead to isolation and loneliness. Negative attitudes can, however, sometimes have a positive effect. Lonsdale (1990) points out that the assumption that disabled women are asexual has advantages and disadvantages; on the one hand it may affect adversely their self-image, but on the other it frees them from sexist expectations. In Morris's book (1989) several of the women interviewed said that disability had liberated their relationships. Vasey can also see advantages, she states:

> We are not usually snapped up in the flower of youth for our domestic and child rearing skills, or for our decorative value, so we do not have to spend years disentangling ourselves from wearisome relationships as is the case with so many non-disabled women. (1992: 74)

Sometimes the change to life an impairment brings is regarded as equally satisfying as life before it occurred. A disabled woman in Morris's book explains:

> As a result of becoming paralysed, life was changed completely. Before my accident it seemed as if I was set to spend the rest of my life as a religious sister but I was not solemnly professed so was not accepted back into the order. Instead I am now very happily married with a home of our own. (1989: 120)

The person who acquires an impairment moves from the role of non-disabled person to disabled person, often very abruptly. It has been suggested that this can give rise to psychological reactions similar to those of the mourning process. Kubler-Ross (1969) presented a five-stage model of psychological adjustment to death and dying. The stages she described were denial, anger, bargaining, depression and acceptance. Burnfield (1985) and many others believe this process to be similar to the psychological reactions required to adjust successfully to acquired impairment. These reactions are by no means inevitable, however, and the assumption that they are has been strongly challenged by Oliver (1983). Silver and Wortman (1980) reviewed the literature on stage models of adaptation after traumatic events and found little evidence to support it. The disabled person may, in fact, report that life has changed for the better, or that difficulties may relate more to social and physical barriers than to the impairment itself. People's reactions to impairment depend on many interacting factors including their personal coping strategies, the kind of life they want to lead, the degree of social support available, the accessibility of the environment and the attitudes and behaviour of others. Lenny (1993) believes that disabled people can sometimes find themselves in a 'catch 22' situation as happiness and contentment following disablement is sometimes viewed as a form of denial.

Many people who acquire an impairment suddenly, however, do report that the experience is profoundly disruptive and disturbing. John Hull (1991) states that he grieved for four-and-a-half years over his lost sight and Maggie, a disabled woman in Campling's book, recalls 'I felt I had little to offer anyone and rather than face rejection, I avoided people. Grieving over the lively gregarious woman I had once been' (1981: 36). Similarly Barbara writes, 'the sense of numbed shock, of powerlessness, anxiety and loss of direction, was my first reasoned response when the realisation that I was partially paralysed penetrated my brain. . . . Anger—a feeling that my body was now flawed, no longer as God meant it to be—and frustration succeeded' (Campling, 1981: 39).

Maggie believes that the intensity of her reaction was probably the result of negative attitudes she had acquired about impairment and disability as a non-disabled person. She states, 'whichever way I turned to think, the negative answer that I was deaf seemed to destroy any shred of hope. I can only think that I learned to expect so little from my future because I somehow soaked up these prevailing attitudes towards women with disabilities as a hearing woman' (Campling, 1981: 35).

It is clear from other accounts of disabled women in Campling's book that those with congenital impairments can also experience a similar psychological upheaval when they grasp the implications of their situation. Michlene recalls the day when she realized she would always be disabled:

> That momentous day I suddenly realised. . . . I was going to be the same as I had always been—very small, funnily shaped, unable to walk. It seemed at that moment that the sky cracked. . . . The next two years seemed like a dark roller-coaster ride, sometimes happy, often plunging into despair. My main preoccupation seemed to be desperately trying to deny the awareness of my difference which had started on that day. (Campling, 1981: 24)

Accounts such as these demonstrate that the notion of people with congenital impairments 'not knowing what they are missing' is untrue, and probably serves the purpose of making non-disabled people feel less guilty and responsible, as well as denying that anything substantial needs to be done to improve the lives of disabled people. It is obvious that visually impaired people *do* know what they are missing as they wait for a bus on a cold, dark night while everyone else gets into their cars, and that physically-disabled people know what they are missing when denied access to the theatre, the library or the public toilet. As Wilkinson puts it, 'The "loss" does not concern what was . . . but what could have been' (1992: 418). It is often said that disabled people have qualities and attributes to compensate for these losses, such as the 'sixth sense' of blind people, the cheerfulness of those with learning difficulties and the bravery of people who use wheelchairs. Such notions are, however, false: disabled people possess the same range of attributes as non-disabled people.

People who acquire impairments frequently experience serious problems with their relationships. Burnfield (1985) mentions that marriages often break down after the onset of multiple sclerosis, especially if they were under strain beforehand. The disabled person may need to build a new self-image, cope with greater dependency on others for everyday needs and change direction in occupation and leisure activities. Shakespeare states:

> A handicap acquired later in life involves a somewhat different type of realisation, in general much more rapid than the realisation of congenital handicap. In this case the self-concept has to be altered and with severe disability a totally new one has to be acquired. Alongside this process, others who knew him before he became handicapped need to get to know him again. People in the position of becoming handicapped in later life generally report that interaction is easier with new acquaintances than with those who were known previous to the handicap. (1975: 20)

To suggest such a profound change in the individual following the onset of impairment is almost certainly exaggerated. Morris (1989) found that for many of the women with spinal-cord injuries she spoke to, life went on much the same as it had before their accident or illness. However, those who acquire an impairment, particularly if its onset is rapid, are probably more likely than those with congenital impairments, or those who develop impairments more slowly, to feel an acute sense of loss and a need to change many aspects of their lives. Because of their past experience as non-disabled people, those who acquire an impairment in adulthood may comprehend their disadvantaged status in society more clearly than those who have always been disabled.

People with progressive impairments must cope continually with altered and diminished bodily function. Even those with static impairments are more affected by the ageing process than their non-disabled peers (Zarb, 1993). Paralysed people, for example, may develop early and severe arthritis in their over-used joints, and partially-sighted and partially-hearing people may be adversely affected by small 'normal' losses in their hearing and sight.

When attempting to assess and respond effectively to the psychological reactions manifested by disabled people, it is important to attempt to distinguish psychological reactions to impairment and disability from psychological reactions resulting from physiological and pathological changes which may be brought about by the disease or injury. Following a stroke or head injury, for example, people may become aggressive, forgetful or depressed. Psychological changes can also occur in diseases such as Parkinson's disease and Huntington's chorea. Sometimes it is the medications people are taking which produce these effects, while the physical and social environment can also have a profound effect on the individual's psychological state. These complex interactions are explored in more detail by Finkelstein and French (1993).

The visibility of the impairment

Various researchers have found that people with a less obvious or hidden impairment have more social difficulties than those with a more visible impairment. This is so even though the less obvious impairment is often less severe in terms of function. Gulliford (1971) found that children with severe impairments were better adjusted than those with less severe impairments, and Cowen and Bobrove (1966) found that both deaf and blind people were better adjusted than partially-hearing and partially-sighted people. The deaf and blind people saw themselves as being less rejected, and were more accepting of themselves than the partially-hearing and partially-sighted people.

Dodds et al. (1992) found partially-sighted adults to have more negative attitudes towards blindness and a lower sense of personal effectiveness than blind adults. White states:

> socially it is tougher to be partially sighted than blind. You are a constant prey to misunderstandings and even accusations of fraud. ('One minute she's tapping along with a white stick; next minute she's gazing into a shop window' or 'I smiled at him and he just walked by as if I wasn't there.') (1990: 11)

Wright (1992) points out the importance of greetings and acknowledgements, such as smiles and waves, and how their absence can have a lasting and negative effect.

Straughair and Fawcitt report similar misunderstandings from their interviews with young people with arthritis. One respondent explained:

> My neighbours are very good but I'm sure they sometimes think I am a fraud. I have trouble getting started in the morning because I am so stiff and I have to send my little girl next door to get the lid off the marmalade jar. But then in the afternoon when the stiffness has gone I go horse-riding. (1992: 49)

Davis (1984) found that the more clearly defined and visible the impairment, the greater the facility with which disabled people and non-disabled people adjust to each other. Albrecht (1982) believes that the major factor in producing social distance between disabled and non-disabled people is the degree of disruption to social interaction. Soder (1991) develops the argument further, suggesting that poor interaction between disabled and non-disabled people is due, not to prejudice on the part of non-disabled people, but to ambivalence. Drewitt (1990) reports that interaction with others became much easier once her impairments could be seen.

Disabled people with hidden impairments are in a position to decide whether or not to reveal them. In every situation they must determine how the impairment will be received, whether or not it is relevant to mention it, how likely it is to be discovered, and what the consequences of that discovery will be. People with more obvious impairments are only free to make such decisions if their communications are not face to face, for example when filling in a form or speaking on the telephone—provided that the impairment does not involve speech and language.

Revealing an impairment or hiding it has the potential for both positive and negative outcomes as illustrated in Figure 2.2.

In reality, hiding an impairment is rarely a positive experience, even if it is never discovered, because the process of hiding it is often very stressful; people cannot ask for what they need and must constantly try to avoid situations where the impairment may be discovered, or be ready with excuses and explanations if it is. The

	Positive outcomes	Negative outcomes
Reveal disability	Disabled person is accepted	Disabled person is rejected
Hide disability	Impairment is never discovered	Impairment is discovered

Figure 2.2

partially-hearing person, for example, may pretend to be absent-minded; the person with slight ataxia, clumsy; and the person with learning difficulties, who finds it hard to cope socially, introverted. A psychological cost is therefore paid for silence. The alternative labels (absent-minded, clumsy etc) are also derogatory but, for the people concerned, less so than their real impairments. An alternative strategy to silence is openness in an attempt to educate others. Scambler (1984) found this a very rare strategy among people with epilepsy.

It is interesting to note that on occasions people may portray themselves as having other, less discrediting, characteristics. In the novel *Judgement in Stone* by Ruth Rendell (1978), for example, Eunice Parchman, who cannot read, pretends to have very poor sight and is in a constant state of anxiety in case her excellent vision and her real limitation are discovered. Similarly those found guilty of crimes may plead 'diminished responsibility' or amnesia as an alternative label to 'criminal'. Sometimes hiding an impairment or limitation becomes so habitual that people start to enact the characteristics of the alternative label. Visually-impaired people who avoid parties and outings in case their impairment is discovered may, over the years, become rather isolated and lacking in social skills. They may gradually start to view themselves as people who prefer to be alone.

Scambler, writing about people with epilepsy, has questioned the degree to which stigma is 'real' rather than 'felt'. He found that only rarely do people's perceptions of their stigmatized condition arise from instances of negative discrimination. He states that 'felt stigma, and especially the fear of enacted stigma, was typically the source of more personal anguish and unhappiness than was enacted stigma' and that 'felt stigma was in its own right a profound and lasting, if intermittent, source of unease, self-doubt and disruption in people's lives' (1984: 217).

Another problem which arises for those with hidden or less obvious impairments or disabilities is that help is not always offered when needed and is frequently inappropriate when given. Those with visible impairments are not entirely free of such problems either, as people are generally poorly informed about impairment and disability whatever its degree (McConkey and McCormack, 1983). However, there must be more potential for people to respond appropriately to a person's impairment if they can see what it is. This can make disguising impairments, for example by using elaborate prostheses, a problem and a psychological burden for some disabled people (Sutherland, 1981).

Given that concealing an impairment is a stressful and difficult process, but is, nonetheless, regarded as the best option by many for whom it is possible, it follows that the problems of having an obvious impairment must be equally bad, or perhaps worse. The difficulty which people with obvious impairments face is the tendency of others immediately to label them 'disabled' with all the misconceptions and stereotypes that the label implies. The impairment is considered to be the person's most important attribute, obscuring all others. This can have serious consequences when trying to find employment, gain acceptance on a college course, or make friends. The reactions of others can also be humiliating and demoralizing. Sue, a disabled woman featured in Campling's book, explains:

> My weak grasp on my identity was no real match for the massed forces of society who firmly believed themselves as 'normal' and myself just as firmly as 'abnormal'. I found myself inhabiting a stereotype. I became my illness. I was of interest only because of it. And as a person in a wheelchair I elicited embarrassment, avoidance, condescension, personal questions. . . . Going out became a nightmare, I was public property. People either staring intently into my face, or looking away. (1981: 48)

It should also be appreciated that many people with obvious impairments also have hidden ones. Take people with paraplegia, for example, although the fact of their paraplegia is obvious, the associated problems of impotence and incontinence, which may be present, are hidden from view. Julie, a disabled woman featured in Campling's book, explains, 'In intimate relationships there is always that first moment when the mechanics of your bladder management are revealed. This is the major test. How will he react to a mature woman who wears plastic knickers, pads and requires help going to the loo?' (1981: 17). Burnfield (1985) speaks of the hidden impairments associated with multiple sclerosis, such as fatigue, blurred vision and sensory disturbances. Problems such as these are frequently misunderstood and made more incomprehensible by their fluctuating nature (Straughair and Fawcitt, 1992).

The situation for people with sporadic impairments, for example those with epilepsy, is rather different; they appear non-disabled most of the time but when their impairment manifests itself it may be either obvious to others or relatively hidden. Despite the fact that 80 per cent of people with epilepsy have the condition totally or well controlled by drugs (British Epilepsy Association), it remains a very stigmatized condition which can lead to an urgent need to conceal it. Hevey (1990) refutes the idea that people with epilepsy are only disabled during their actual seizures, believing that the terror and fear of epilepsy, born of other people's reactions, can render people with epilepsy 'epileptics' all the time.

The comprehensibility of the impairment and disability to others

The functional ability of disabled people is often markedly affected by the situation they are in. Partially-hearing people, for example, may only understand speech in an environment free from background noise, and with voices of a certain pitch. They may communicate well on the telephone but not in social situations, be able to hear the voices of men but not women and find voices too loud even though they cannot understand what is being said. Their situation is perhaps less easy to understand than that of profoundly-deaf people who may not hear speech whatever the circumstance. Partially-sighted people may function entirely differently according to the lighting; rushing around confidently in overcast conditions but needing to be guided on bright sunny days, or vice versa (French, 1988). Similarly people with heart complaints may use wheelchairs on some occasions but not on others.

These ambiguities can even make it difficult for disabled people to comprehend fully their own situation, especially when the impairment has been recently acquired. Dodds et al. explain:

> The partially sighted clients we spoke to mentioned that they had difficulty in trying to make other people understand their disability. This is understandable, as partial sight can be very confusing to the sufferer as well as the onlooker. For example, a client who can read a newspaper but who is unable to move through the environment without using a cane may feel, as well as appear to be, a fraud . . . the totally blind client can more easily fulfil a well established set of non-visual expectations. (1992: 294)

Because the functional ability of disabled people varies so much according to environmental circumstances, their situation is difficult to comprehend. This is a particular problem for those with relatively hidden impairments, although there is much confusion surrounding more obvious impairments too. The blind person, or the person with an unsteady gait, for example, are likely to function more competently in a familiar setting, and the person using a wheelchair will be less disabled in surroundings suited to his or her needs. The social and psychological environment must also be considered: the deaf person may cope with communication better if the atmosphere is friendly and supportive, and the person with a tremor may find that anxiety or lack of time tends to make it worse. All of these factors have major implications when assessing disabled people.

Because of the ambiguous nature of impairment and disability, the behaviour of disabled people is often interpreted in terms of intellectual or personality deficits. For example the child with slight ataxia may be reprimanded for being careless, or teased for being clumsy, or the partially-hearing person, who fails to reply, may be considered hostile and unfriendly. Shearer (1981) quotes a man with multiple sclerosis who found people kind and generous when he was eventually compelled to use a wheelchair, but before his disease progressed to that stage they usually thought he was drunk. The man seen to read a newspaper on the ward who insists that he needs help to find his way to an adjoining hospital block, the deaf person who can hear what the doctor says but not the nurse, and the woman with a motor impairment who manages to walk in the ward but insists that she cannot walk outside, are probably not being 'awkward' at all; at least that is only one of several possible explanations.

To complicate the situation still further, impairments placed within the same category or arising from the same condition or disease rarely produce identical manifestations. These manifestations can, in fact, be extremely diverse. Thus one partially-sighted person may be able to see colour and rely on it a great deal, while another may be colour blind; the first person may function best in bright light but the second when the light is dim (French, 1988). People with epilepsy have different types of fits, and the manifestations of those with head injury, or people diagnosed as having multiple sclerosis, can be entirely different. Further ambiguities and confusion can arise because conditions and diseases, which are not particularly similar, are often confused, for example learning difficulties and mental illness, rheumatoid arthritis and osteoarthritis, nervous disease and psychiatric illness.

The manifestations of impairment are poorly understood and tend to be individualized. This is epitomized in the notion that disabled people with less severe disabilities have an inner identity crisis, not knowing whether to associate with disabled or non-disabled people. As Shakespeare states:

> A basic dilemma of the handicapped person is that of which group he belongs to, whether he should identify himself with 'the handicapped' or to what extent he should consider himself part of normal society. He finds he is a member of society but different from most other members. Hence he is often unsure where he belongs . . . it has been suggested that the severely handicapped experience less stress here, as they are

clearly handicapped and have fewer opportunities of choice. The psychological position of the less severely handicapped has been referred to as 'marginality', as they are between total disability and normality. (1975: 25)

Although some disabled people may believe this to be true, the roots of the problem almost certainly lie in the responses of non-disabled people, who cannot understand or cope with the complexities and ambiguities of disability (Ryan and Thomas, 1987; Ozer, 1990). Shaw notes that when she tries to explain her disability, it is seen as 'embarrassing moaning', but when she keeps quiet about it people protest that they cannot help her if she will not inform them (1990: 15). Hevey found that every time he attempted to 'come out' about his epilepsy he was silenced and found himself capitulating. He realized that 'the hidden power contract was to stay like "us" or be obliterated' (1992: 79).

The presence or absence of illness

Many disabled people are extremely fit and healthy, but for others their impairment is associated with illness. Illness can be defined as the subjective feeling of being unwell and may include symptoms of pain, breathlessness, tiredness and vertigo. Some conditions which may give rise to impairment, for example, rheumatoid arthritis and glaucoma, are associated with considerable pain. Pain, particularly when prolonged, has the potential to cause anxiety and depression. This can give rise to a viscious circle as both states of mind tend to heighten the perception of pain (French, 1992b). Bond states, 'Pain, especially if chronic, brings feelings of depression and those that become depressed easily may not only sink emotionally but simultaneously experience more pain . . . at the same time they show reduced ability to cope with it' (1984: 46).

Prolonged pain, even if not particularly severe, tends to take the joy out of life. Even activities which previously seemed exciting may become dull and uninteresting (Peck, 1982). This lack of activity means that time can hang heavily and depression may intensify. Peck (1982) believes that feelings of having little control over the situation also contribute to depression. Davison and Neale (1990) point out that anxiety and depression frequently co-exist.

Pain is intrusive and the people who experience it may find it very difficult to concentrate on anything properly or cope with physical or social demands. They may mix with other people less, and have little to talk about, or talk only about their pain. In time their company may become less rewarding to others who may withdraw or cope with the situation by denying the reality of the pain. Peck (1982) believes that this can lead to a cycle of resentment and guilt, as well as feelings of anger and irritability on the part of both the people experiencing pain and their families and friends.

Morris, in her book about the experiences of women with spinal-cord injuries, devotes an entire chapter to the subject of pain. She states:

> One in four of us experience pain which is so serious that it curtails our activities or confines us to bed for all or part of the time. Pain does not seem to follow any set pattern for any particular level of lesion, whether cervical, thoracic or lumbar, or whether complete or incomplete. (1989: 176)

Anita, who is featured in this book, complains that:

> The common reaction from professionals and lay people is: 'If you can't feel, how can you have pain?' This is very upsetting. Most professionals know about the phantom pain amputees suffer, so why can they not accept that we have a great deal of pain, even though there may be no sensory feeling? (1989: 177)

Disabled people who cope with pain as well as disability are clearly in a very different position to people who, though severely disabled, are free of pain.

Another symptom of illness is extreme fatigue which is felt, for example, by many people with multiple sclerosis. Burnfield (1985) reports on a Canadian survey of people with multiple sclerosis where it was found that fatigue was the most distressing symptom for 40 per cent of the respondents. Fatigue is, of course, relatively hidden, which can lead to a lack of understanding and belief. Burnfield (1985) reveals that his wife thought he was trying to avoid working in the garden when he complained that he was tired. Sexual relationships, social life and work may all be adversely affected. Fatigue may also arise because of the effort required to function with an impairment. Dodds explains that visual impairment 'involves the person in a lot of effort. Great amounts of concentration are required to extract useful information and this is tiring' (1993: 149).

Breathlessness, associated with conditions such as asthma and bronchitis, may also give rise to psychological and social problems. Rubeck interviewed people with chronic bronchitis and found that many of them reported fear of choking or suffocation. One person said 'your shoulders try to meet in front of you, tighter and tighter . . . you think you're going to choke . . . you gasp and gasp to get your breath, and then you panic' (1971: 26). Morgan et al. (1983) found that the anxiety level of people with bronchitis was more predictive of their ability to walk a given distance than the function of their lungs. Most nurses and therapists will have treated patients or clients who are far more disabled by this type of fear than they are by their actual impairments.

As well as understanding the situation of disabled people who have symptoms of illness, it is vitally important to recognize that many disabled people are as fit and as free from symptoms as anyone else. Not only are impairment and disability frequently unassociated with illness, but there is often no link with a disease process either. The belief that disability is inevitably linked to severe illness and disease has given rise to many misconceptions about disabled people with far-reaching effects such as reluctance to employ them.

Conclusion

In the last analysis, disabled people are individuals who respond to their situation in unique ways. However, by considering the dimensions of impairment and disability presented in this chapter, it is possible to gain a greater understanding of the difficulties and barriers disabled people face. Other factors, such as whether or not the condition is progressive, how certain the prognosis is, the gender and social class of the individual, and how acceptable the impairment is to others, can also provide valuable insights. Without this knowledge there will be a lack of understanding between health professionals, such as therapists and nurses, and disabled people, which will inevitably interfere with the success of treatment and rehabilitation.

References

Albrecht, G. (1982) Social distance from the stigmatised: a test of two theories. *Social Science and Medicine*, **16**, 1319–27

Bond, M. R. (1984) *Pain: Its Nature, Analysis and Treatment*, 2nd edn, Churchill Livingstone, London

Brudenell, P. (1986) *The Other Side of Profound Handicap*, Macmillan, London

Burlington, D. (1979) To be blind in a sighted world. *Psychoanalytic Study of the Child*, **34**, 5–30

Burnfield, A. (1985) *Multiple Sclerosis: A Personal Exploration*, Souvenir Press, London

Campling, J. (ed.) (1981) *Images of Ourselves: Women with Disabilities Talking*, Routledge and Kegan Paul, London

Cowen, E. L. and Bobrove, P. H. (1966) Marginality of disability and adjustment. *Perceptual and Motor Skills*, **23 (5)**, 869–870

Davis, S. (1984) Deviance disavowal: the management of strained interaction by the visibly handicapped. In *The Other Side*, (ed. H. Becker), Free Press, Illinois

Davison, G. C. and Neale, J. M. (1990) *Abnormal Psychology*, 5th edn, John Wiley & Sons, New York

Dodds, A. G. (1993) *Rehabilitating Blind and Visually Impaired People*, Chapman & Hall, London

Dodds, A. G., Ng, L. and Yates, L. (1992) Residential rehabilitation 1: client characteristics. *The New Beacon*, **76 (901)**, 321–325

Drewitt, J. (1990) Disabilities no-one can see. *Disability Now*, November, 11

Finkelstein, V. and French, S. (1993) Towards a psychology of disability. In *Disabling Barriers—Enabling Environments*, (eds J. Swain, V. Finkelstein, S. French and M. Oliver), Sage, London

French, S. (1988) Understanding partial sight. *Nursing Times*, **83 (3)**, 32–33

French, S. (1992a) Ageism. In *Physiotherapy: A Psychosocial Approach*, (ed. S. French), Butterworth-Heinemann, Oxford

French, S. (1992b) The psychology and sociology of pain. In *Physiotherapy: A Psychosocial Approach*, (ed. S. French), Butterworth-Heinemann, Oxford

Gulliford, R. (1971) *Special Educational Needs*, Routledge & Kegan Paul, London

Hevey, D. (1990) Hidden disabilities: help or hindrance? *Disability Now*, October, 14–15

Hevey, D. (1992) *The Creatures Time Forgot: Photography and Disability Imagery*, Routledge, London

Hull, J. (1991) *Touching the Rock: An Experience of Blindness*, Arrow Books, London

Kubler-Ross, E. (1969) *On Death and Dying*, Tavistock Publications, London

Lenny, J. (1993) Do disabled people need counselling? In *Disabling Barriers—Enabling Environments*, (eds J. Swain, V. Finkelstein, S. French and M. Oliver), Sage, London

Lewis, V. (1987) *Development and Handicap*, Basil Blackwell, Oxford

Lonsdale, S. (1990) *Women and Disability*, Macmillan, London

McConkey, R. and McCormack, B. (1983) *Breaking Barriers: Educating People about Disability*, Souvenir Press, London

Morgan, A., Peck, D. and Buchaman, D. (1983) Psychological factors in chronic bronchitis. *British Medical Journal*, **286**, 171–173

Morris, J. (1989) *Able Lives*, The Women's Press, London

Murphy, F. M. and O'Driscoll, M. (1989) Observation of the motor development of visually impaired children. *Physiotherapy*, **75 (9)**, 505–508

Oliver, M. (1983) *Social Work and Disabled People*, Macmillan, London

Oswin, M. (1978) *Holes in the Welfare Net*, Bedford Square Press, London

Ozer, L. (1990) Hidden disability. In *Perspectives on Disability*, (M. Nagler), Health Markets Research, Palo Alto, California

Peck, C. (1982) *Controlling Chronic Pain*, Fontana, London

Rendell, R. (1978) *A Judgement in Stone*, Arrow Books, London

Rubeck, M. F. (1971) *Social and Emotional Effects of Chronic Bronchitis*, Health Horizon Limited, London

Ryan, J. and Thomas, F. (1987) *The Politics of Mental Handicap*, Free Association Books, London

Scambler, G. (1984) Perceiving and coping with stigmatising illness. In *The Experience of Illness*, (eds R. Fitzpatrick, J. Hinton, S. Newman et al.), Tavistock Publications, London

Shakespeare, R. (1975) *The Psychology of Handicap*, Methuen, London

Shaw, G. (1990) Hidden disabilities: help or hindrance? *Disability Now*, October, 14–15

Shearer, A. (1980) *Handicapped Children in Residential Care*, Bedford Square Press, London

Shearer, A. (1981) *Disability: Whose Handicap?* Basil Blackwell, Oxford

Silver, R. L. and Wortman, C. B. (1980) Coping with undesirable events. In *Human Helplessness*, (eds J. Garber and M. E. P. Seligman), Academic Press, New York

Soder, M. (1991) Prejudice or ambivalence? Attitudes towards persons with disabilities. *Disability, Handicap and Society*, **5 (3)**, 227–242

Straughair, S. and Fawcitt, S. (1992) *The Road Towards Independence: The Experiences of Young People with Arthritis in the 1990s*, Arthritis Care, London

Sutherland, A. T. (1981) *Disabled We Stand*, Souvenir Press, London

Vasey, S. (1992) Disability culture: it's a way of life. In *Disability Equality in the Classroom: A Human Rights Issue*, (R. Rieser and M. Mason), Disability Equality in Education, London

Walker, J. A. and Crawley, S. B. (1983) Conceptual and methodological issues in studying the handicapped infant. In *Educating Handicapped Infants: Issues in Development and Intervention*, (eds S. Gray Garwood and R. R. Fewell), Aspen Systems Corporation, Rockville

White, P. (1990) Disabilities no-one can see. *Disability Now*, November, 11

Wilkinson, H. (1992) A step out of denial. *The New Beacon*, **76 (903)**, 418–419

Wright, B. (1992) *Communication Skills*, Churchill Livingstone, Edinburgh

Zarb, G. (1993) The dual experience of ageing with a disability. In *Disabling Barriers—Enabling Environments* (eds J. Swain, V. Finkelstein, S. French and M. Oliver), Sage, London

3

Images of disability

Colin Barnes

Introduction

This chapter focuses on stereotypical portrayals of disabled people in the media and shows how they nurture and perpetuate negative assumptions about impairment and disability. Although the misrepresentation of disability in charity advertising is of particular concern to disabled people and their organizations, it deals with the media as a whole. The discussion does not cover specialist disability media, often controlled and run by disabled people themselves, which usually provide a positive alternative. Examples include BBC television's *Close to the Edge*, ITV's *Link* programme, Derbyshire Coalition of Disabled People's *Info* or Greater Manchester Coalition of Disabled People's quarterly magazine *Coalition*. It is divided into two parts: the first part focuses upon institutional discrimination against disabled people and the role of the media, and the second examines commonly recurring media stereotypes of disabled people.

Institutional discrimination and the media

There is now clear evidence from several sources that Britain's 6.5 million disabled people experience a lifestyle of poverty and dependency (Barnes, 1991; Berthoud et al., 1993; Martin et al., 1988).

Traditional medical explanations suggest this is because impairment has such a traumatic physical and psychological effect on individuals that they are unable to achieve a comparable lifestyle to non-disabled people by their own efforts. Disabled people and their organizations reject this as a sound basis for understanding the problems associated with disability (Finkelstein, 1980; Oliver, 1990; Sutherland, 1981).

They, along with a growing number of professionals and policy makers, particularly from overseas, maintain that it is not 'impairment'—individually-based functional limitations whether physical, sensory, intellectual or hidden—which prevents people from achieving a reasonable lifestyle, but restrictive environments and disabling barriers. Thus, 'disability' represents a complex system of social constraints imposed on people with impairments by a highly discriminatory society.

The problem is compounded for disabled members of the lesbian and gay communities, disabled black people, disabled women and disabled members of other marginalized groupings (Begum, 1992; Killin, 1993; Lonsdale, 1990; Morris, 1991). This is because in addition to discrimination on the grounds of impairment they also encounter other forms of institutional prejudice such as heterosexism, racism and sexism (see chapters 13 and 15).

The type of discrimination experienced by disabled people is not simply a question of individual prejudice, though this is a common view, it is institutionalized in the very fabric of our society. Recent research shows that institutional discrimination—attitudes and policies which deny basic human rights and equal opportunities to disabled people—is evident in education, the labour market, the benefit system, health and support services, the built environment, the leisure industry and the media (Barnes, 1991).

Stereotypical assumptions about disabled people are based on superstition, myths and beliefs from earlier, less enlightened times. They are inherent to our culture and persist partly because they are constantly reproduced through the communications media. We learn about disability from the media and in the same way that racist or sexist attitudes, whether implicit or explicit, are acquired through the 'normal' learning process, so too are negative assumptions about disabled people.

While the media alone cannot be held responsible for this situation, its impact should not be underestimated. Official figures show that 98 per cent of British homes have a television, and on average we spend at least 24¾ hours a week watching it. Sixty-five per cent of the population read a daily newspaper, 72 per cent a Sunday newspaper, 9 per cent read magazines and 81 per cent of the 26 per cent who use public libraries borrow books (HMSO, 1991). Whilst there is some dispute about the influence the media has on our perceptions of the world there are few who believe it has none. There is, for example, widespread public concern about the long-term effects of broadcasting and the media on children (BSC, 1989).

Commonly recurring media stereotypes

The link between impairment and all that is socially unacceptable was first established in classical Greek theatre (Hevey, 1992). Today there are several cultural stereotypes which perpetuate this linkage (Barnes, 1992; Biklen and Bogdana, 1977; Gartner and Joe, 1987). But these depictions are not necessarily mutually exclusive, frequently one will be linked to another. The disabled person as evil, for example, is often combined with the disabled person as sexually degenerate. The point is that the overall view of disabled people is decidedly negative and a threat to the non-disabled community.

Probably the most common disabling stereotype is the disabled person as pitiable and pathetic. A view recently advanced by the growth of TV charity shows such as *Comic Relief*, *Children in Need* and *Telethon*—programmes which encourage pity and sentimentality so that non-disabled people can feel bountiful. It is a regular feature of popular fiction, in which overtly dependent disabled people are included in storylines to depict another character's goodness and sensitivity.

Disabled individuals are often portrayed as especially endearing to elicit even greater feelings of sentimentality; their well-being dependent solely upon the benevolence of others. This is a recurrent theme in *all* media depictions of disability. Well-known examples include Tiny Tim in Charles Dickens's *Christmas Carol*, and Porgy in George Gershwin's opera *Porgy and Bess* (Reiser, 1992).

This entirely negative view of disabled people appears regularly both on television and in the press. Pictures of disabled individuals, frequently children, in hospitals or in nursing homes, are repeatedly flashed across our TV screens perpetuating the misconception that disability is synonymous with illness and suffering. Research shows that most reports about disabled people in TV news programmes and documentaries are about medical treatments and impairment-related cures (Cumberbatch and Negrine, 1992). Besides stimulating sympathy, this constant repetition of the medical approach to impairment helps to divert the public's attention away from the social factors which create disability (see chapter 1).

Moreover, the language used in these emotive broadcasts creates a mood of sentimentality which is both patronizing and offensive to disabled people. While many reporters use acceptable terminology such as 'disabled people' their reports still have an overtly sentimental tone because they insist on referring to disabled individuals as 'plucky', 'brave', 'courageous', 'victims', 'sufferers' or 'unfortunate'. Such terms say more about the value judgements of the reporters themselves than they do about the experience of disability. Derogatory words like 'cripple' or 'dummies' are never used but TV news stories often include impersonal expressions such as 'the disabled' and 'the handicapped'—phrases which offend because they rob disabled people of their humanity, and so reduce them to objects (see French, 1989).

News stories about health and about fundraising events depicting disabled people as pitiable, passive and dependent regularly crop up in British newspapers—accounting for about two thirds of all coverage (Smith and Jordan, 1991). In many cases these reports are grossly inaccurate and damaging to disabled people. Journalists frequently patronize disabled people by referring to them by their first name rather than by their full title as they do in stories about non-disabled people.

In spite of the well-publicized concern among the disabled community about the tactics used by charity advertisers, they still portray disabled people in this way in order to raise money. Impairment-specific organizations like Mencap, The Muscular Dystrophy Group, and The Multiple Sclerosis Society regularly present this view of disabled people in a variety of forms: in cinemas, on television, in the press and in the deluge of unwanted 'junk mail' which most of us receive through our letter boxes (Hevey, 1992).

By emphasizing the 'tragedy' of disability these advertisements perpetuate the inaccurate assumption that living with impairment is a life-shattering experience. This effectively robs some disabled individuals of the self-confidence to overcome disability. They also cultivate the notion that disabled people have something 'wrong' with them and so maintain the social barriers between them and non-disabled people. Furthermore, the constant repetition of traditional medical explanations of disability by organizations which in the public mind have disabled people's best interests at heart seriously undermines the environmental approach favoured by disabled people themselves. In short, rather than alleviate disabled people's dependency these advertisements promote it.

Throughout history disabled people have been the victims of violence. The ancient Greeks and the Romans were enthusiastic advocates of infanticide for disabled children. In medieval Europe disability was associated with evil and witchcraft and in some areas the persecution and murder of disabled people was approved by religious leaders. During the nineteenth century scientific legitimacy for violence against disabled people was provided by the theories of Charles Darwin and the eugenics movement. Eugenic ideals reached their climax during the 1939-45 war with the systematic murder of approximately 80–100,000 disabled people by the German Nazi party. There remains tacit support for these ideas among sections of the general population; notably among supporters of neo- fascist organizations such as the National Front and the British National Party.

The absence in literature and other media of a full range of roles for disabled people cultivates assumptions that disabled people are defenceless and susceptible to violence. The portrayal of disabled people as victims of violence is common in films and on television. The Hollywood classics *Woman in a Cage* and *Whatever Happened to Baby Jane* are both fine examples. In the former, Olivia de Haviland, a wheelchair user, is trapped in a lift by a gang of young thugs while they ransack her flat. In the latter, Joan Crawford, also a wheelchair user, is abused by her murderous sister, Bette Davis.

Newspapers often sensationalize violence against disabled people. For example, one study found that over half the stories about people with learning difficulties in the national and local press portrayed them as victims. The extent of this victimization included sexual and physical abuse, theft and vandalism (Wertheimer, 1988). Besides nurturing the idea that disabled people are helpless, pitiable and unable to survive without protection, these stories emphasize, albeit implicitly, the eugenic conviction that the natural solution to the problem of impairment is a violent one.

The association between impairment and evil is one of the most persistent stereotypes and a major obstacle to disabled people's successful integration into the community. The classic example is Shakespeare's *Richard III*. Exploiting early beliefs about physical impairment—in the Bible there are over forty instances in which 'the cripple' is connected to sin and sinners—Shakespeare portrays Richard as twisted in both body and mind. Similar distortions are common in literature and art—both classical and popular.

Writers of children's books have exploited this stereotype to the hilt: Stevenson's *Treasure Island* is a good example. In evoking the terror and suspense that mark the book's opening pages the key elements are the disabled characters Black Dog and Blind Pew. The former is introduced as 'a sallow faced man wanting two fingers' and the latter as 'a hunched and eyeless creature', and it is Pew who hands Billy Bones the dread black spot.

The depiction of disabled people as evil is a particular favourite among filmmakers. The list of films which connect impairment to wickedness and villainy is virtually endless. *Dr Jekyll and Mr Hyde* symbolizes the stark contrast between goodness and evil; Dr Jekyll is straight backed, handsome and virtuous while his alter ego, Mr Hyde, is hunched, ugly and 'mad'. Other memorable examples include the maniacal and multi-impaired Peter Sellers in *Dr Strangelove*, the villains in *Dirty Harry* and *The Sting*—all of whom limped—and the profusion of disabled criminals in the James Bond films. Additionally, fictional programmes on television often portray disabled people as criminals or monsters.

Similar themes regularly appear in the press. Newspaper articles sensationalizing the connection between intellectual impairments and criminality are common in both the tabloids and the 'quality' papers (Wertheimer, 1988). The overall message coming out of these stories is that such people cannot be trusted, are a danger to children and should be locked up.

Such imagery is grossly inaccurate and does much harm to public perceptions of people with intellectual impairments and, by implication, the disabled community as a whole. In general they are more likely to be introverted and sensitive than violent and aggressive, they are more likely to avoid rather than attack others, and given the appropriate support they are perfectly capable of living in the community.

Disabled people are sometimes included in the storylines of films and TV dramas to enhance a certain atmosphere, usually one of menace, mystery or deprivation, or to add character to the visual impact of the production. This dilutes the humanity of disabled people by reducing them to objects of curiosity. Take for instance the classic horror film *Frankenstein* starring Boris Karloff. To amplify the overall sense of menace the filmmakers included a 'hunchback', Fritz, as Baron Frankenstein's only servant. The character does not appear in Mary Shelley's original novel. Fritz's role in the film is also significant because he is presented as ultimately responsible for the monster's evil ways rather than its creator—the non-disabled Baron.

In the early part of the film, when Frankenstein is creating the monster, he sends Fritz to fetch a particular brain to be placed in its skull. While completing this task Fritz carelessly drops the brain, damaging it beyond repair, and then substitutes another—one taken from a known criminal. Later as the plot unfolds and the monster's true nature becomes apparent Fritz taunts it with a blazing torch, thus causing it to embark on its murderous rampage—the Baron appears relatively blameless.

Disabled individuals are sometimes represented as 'super cripples'. This is similar to the stereotype portrayal of black people as having 'super' qualities in order to elicit respect from white people. Black people are often depicted as having 'a wonderful sense of rhythm', or as exceptional athletes. With disability, however, the disabled person is assigned super-human almost magical abilities. Blind people are portrayed as visionaries with a sixth sense or extremely sensitive hearing. Alternatively, disabled individuals, especially children, are praised excessively for relatively ordinary achievements.

Although there are many examples of the super-cripple film one of best known is the award winning *My Left Foot*. Based on the disabled writer and artist Christy Brown's autobiography—he referred to it as 'my plucky little cripple story'—it tells the tale of how Brown 'overcomes' both impairment and the poverty of working-class life in Dublin in the 1930s to become nationally acclaimed as an artist, writer and poet. The familiar theme that disabled people's achievements are dependent on the benevolence of others is also strongly represented in this film. It is as much about the strong support network of women surrounding Brown as it is about Brown himself, notably his mother who refused to believe the doctors when they told her Christy was a vegetable, the doctor whose belief in him played an important part in his 'rehabilitation' and the nurse who fell in love with him.

Similar themes abound in news stories about disabled people's achievements—either extraordinary or managing to fit into a 'normal life'—both on television and in the press. On television they account for over a quarter of all news stories about disabled people. A high proportion of these reports are charity appeals like *Children in Need* or emotive shows like *Hearts of Gold*. The mood of these broadcasts is predictably sympathetic and heart-rending with statements such as 'These children have shown talent and determination in overcoming their disabilities' (Cumberbatch and Negrine, 1992). This triumph over tragedy approach precludes the crucial point that disability is a social issue which cannot be addressed by misplaced sentimentality over individual impairments.

The cartoon character Mr Magoo, an elderly man with visual impairment, epitomizes society's perceptions of the disabled person as the hapless fool. Ignorant of his impairment Magoo stumbles through life wreaking havoc, unaware of the innumerable dangers surrounding him although he survives them all. Moreover, throughout Magoo's exploits the audience is constantly reminded that his survival is due to luck rather than his resourcefulness. But laughing at people with impairments is not new, disabled people have been a source of amusement for non-disabled people for centuries. During the seventeenth and eighteenth centuries keeping 'idiots' as objects of humour was quite common, and visits to Bedlam and other institutions were a typical form of entertainment for the able but ignorant.

While such thoughtless behaviour might be expected in earlier, less enlightened times, making fun of disabled people is as prevalent now as it was then. Today the mockery of disabled people is a major feature of many comedy films and TV shows. Take, for instance, the award-winning *A Fish Called Wanda*—one of the film's main characters is an incompetent crook with a severe speech impairment called Ken. Those who exploit this kind of material are not confined to one specific brand of comedy—they are common to them all. The well-known 'establishment' writer and comedian Ronnie Barker, for example, mimicked disabled individuals in two of his most successful TV sit coms: *Clarence*, about an odd-job cum removal man with a visual impairment and *Open All Hours*, about a grocer with a speech impairment.

The negative implications for disabled people of this type of abuse should not be underestimated. First, it seriously undermines what few opportunities they have to be taken seriously by non-disabled society. Second, it has the capacity to sap their self-confidence and esteem. This is especially the case for disabled children as parents of such children are only too aware.

Of course some people might suggest that all sections of the community are sometimes the butt of popular humour and that disabled people cannot and should not expect to be excluded from it. But being mocked publicly is only acceptable if the negative images which ensue can be offset against positive ones, or if those being ridiculed are able to defend themselves should they choose to do so. At present there are virtually no positive images of disabled people in the media, and disabled people do not have the resources or a legal framework within which to fight this type of discrimination.

The media sometimes portray disabled individuals as self-pitiers, who could overcome their difficulties if they would stop feeling sorry for themselves, think positively and rise to 'the challenge' (Biklen and Bogdana, 1977)—a perception which is perhaps not uncommon among health professionals. This is a recurrent theme in many of the so-called 'disability' films produced over the last few years. Well-known examples are *Coming Home* and *Born on The Fourth of July*. Both document the 'psychological trauma' of coming to terms with disability in an able-bodied world. In both films the hero is saved by heterosexual relationships—this was generally considered a step in the right direction because hitherto most 'disability' films depicted disabled people as sexually inactive (see below).

Similar themes sometimes appear in the news media. This is particularly evident with reference to people with HIV and AIDS who have been widely portrayed as solely responsible for their condition. Further, on the few occasions when the press report disabled people campaigning for equal rights they invariably suggest that the campaign might be counter-productive. Following a recent demonstration by CAT (The Campaign for Accessible Transport) in which nine disabled demonstrators were arrested for obstructing traffic one newspaper warned 'Even though the most militant within the disabled lobby can rely on public opinion for their cause. . . . Such tactics will eventually alienate the public support on which the disabled have to rely' (Smith and Jordan, 1991).

Such views stem directly from the traditional medical view of disability. The individual assumptions at the heart of this approach lead to a psychology of impairment which interprets disabled people's behaviour as individual pathology. It allows able-bodied society to reinterpret disabled people's legitimate anger over disablism as self-destructive bitterness arising out of an inability to accept the 'limitations' of impairment. It helps them to avoid addressing the true cause of that anger; ie the attitudes and policies of an overtly disablist society. Hence, in the same way that lesbians, gay men, black people and women are blamed for homophobia, racism and sexism, so too disabled people are blamed for disablism.

Disabled people are often presented as a burden both to their families and to society. During the 1930s the German Third Reich exploited this image extensively in propaganda films justifying their 'euthanasia' programme. In these films disabled people were dehumanized, described as 'Existence Without Life', and presented as an unnecessary burden which must be got rid of (Without Walls, 1991). Similar imagery is present in the media today.

One of the most powerful examples shown on British television was the play *Keeping Tom Nice*, first shown on 15 August 1990. Written by an ex-social worker, it is the story of a family driven to breaking point after 'caring' for their disabled son Tom for twenty-four years. The strain of having a 'vegetable' for a son causes Tom's father to physically abuse him. The fear of being found out by Tom's social worker—who unsurprisingly is portrayed as someone who knows what's best for Tom—leads to his suicide. The play could only have increased viewers' sympathy for families with a similar 'burden', there was nothing in it to evoke empathy with disabled people whatsoever.

This stereotype is connected to the view that disabled people are helpless and must be 'cared' for by non-disabled people. It fails to acknowledge that with appropriate support people with impairments are able to achieve the same level of autonomy and independence as non-disabled people. It comes from the notion that disabled people's needs are profoundly different to those of the non-disabled community, and that meeting those needs is an unacceptable drain on society's resources.

Misguided presumptions about disabled people's sexuality have also been a recurrent theme in literature and art since ancient times. The vast majority of these images are about male experiences—there has been little if any exploration of disabled women's sexuality. The disabled writer Louis Battye referred to this stereotype as 'the Chatterly syndrome' following D. H. Lawrence's novel *Lady Chatterly's Lover* (Battye, 1966). The book is about a heterosexual affair between a non-disabled couple: Lady Chatterly and a gamekeeper, Mellors. The relationship takes place because Lady Chatterly's husband is a disabled person, and perceived by Lawrence as sexually inactive.

The perception of disabled women as asexual is particularly pervasive in the media and frequently presented as the perfect alibi for men's adultery. This is a common theme in literature and on television. Take for example Marilyn French's *Bleeding Heart*, a book about an illicit affair between a non-disabled man and a woman—the relationship is justified throughout because the man's wife has an impairment and is incapable of sex. In two recent BBC television dramas *Goodbye Cruel World* and *A Time to Dance* non-disabled men had adulterous affairs because their wives had impairments. Such depictions can only lower the status of disabled women; a status which is already disproportionately undervalued due to the widespread misconception that they are unable to fulfil women's traditional roles of wife and mother.

A variation on this theme is the depiction of the disabled person as sex starved or sexually degenerate. *The Hunchback of Notre Dame* is the classic example. Rejected, isolated and ridiculed by French society, the hunchback, Quasimodo, develops an unhealthy lust for the virginal Esmeralda. Following her rejection he terrorizes the local community until finally he is killed. Sadly, the same story is repeated over and over again in a variety of forms. Moreover, as noted above, the connection between 'mental illness' and sexual perversion is a regular feature of the news media—particularly in the tabloid press.

Finally, disabled people are rarely shown as integral and productive members of the community; as students, as teachers, as part of the workforce or as parents. This feeds the notion that disabled people are inferior human beings with little to offer the community. Apart from the misrepresentations mentioned above, disabled people are conspicuous by their absence from mainstream culture. In TV films and dramas, for example, they represent less than 1½ per cent of all characters portrayed (Cumberbatch and Negrine, 1992). This contrasts dramatically with government evidence showing that at least 12 per cent of the British population are disabled people. Disabled people seldom appear in non-fiction programmes apart from those dealing solely with disability. Moreover, there are no disabled newsreaders, weathermen and women, or presenters of documentaries, and disabled people are hardly ever seen on chat shows in discussions about subjects which do not relate directly to disability.

The exclusion of disabled people from community life is seldom discussed in charity advertising. Few charities, for example, mention disabled people's lack of rights in their advertising campaigns. One of the few exceptions is the recent poster by the Spastics Society depicting a close-up of two babies. Below it is the caption 'One has Cerebral Palsy The Other has Full Human Rights'. Below this is an explicit description of the impairments associated with cerebral palsy, the reason the child is treated differently, the statement 'In an Ideal World She'd turn to the Law, In Reality She'll Turn to the Spastics Society', a description of how the Spastics Society will help—physiotherapy, work experience and training in segregated centres and colleges run by the Spastics Society—and a coupon for donations.

Clearly, apart from the reference to the lack of rights, the message is a familiar one. Impairment—cerebral palsy—is the cause of the problem—unequal treatment—and it can be solved only by solutions which focus on individual disabled people, and not on society. Most importantly, it implies that disabled people have no choice but to turn to charities controlled and run by non-disabled people for help. This is simply not true. Throughout Britain there is a growing network of self-help organizations controlled and run by disabled people themselves providing an alternative approach (see chapter 6). Most of these organizations operate with inadequate funding and little public recognition and support. This and similar commercials effectively deny them that recognition and support. In short, they effectively impede disabled people's struggle for self-determination and independence.

Conclusion

This chapter has demonstrated how the vast majority of information about disability in the mass media is extremely negative. Disabling stereotypes which medicalize, patronize, criminalize and dehumanize disabled people abound in books, films, on television and in the press. They form the bedrock on which the attitudes towards, assumptions about and expectations of disabled people are based. They are fundamental to the discrimination and exploitation which disabled people encounter daily, and contribute significantly to their systematic exclusion from mainstream society. There has been little in the education of health professionals which has counteracted this view. The only solution with any hope of success is for all media organizations to provide the kind of information and imagery which, firstly, acknowledges and explores the complexity of the disability experience and, secondly, facilitates the meaningful integration of *all* disabled people into the economic and social life of the community. Failure to adopt such an approach has important implications for both disabled people and society as a whole.

References

Barnes, C. (1991) *Disabled People in Britain and Discrimination: A Case For Anti-Discrimination Legislation,* C Hurst and Co., London, in Association with the British Council of Organisations of Disabled People

Barnes, C. (1992) *Disabling Imagery and the Media,* Belper, Ryburn in Association with the British Council of Organisations of Disabled People

Begum, N. (1992) *Something to be Proud of. . . . The Lives of Asian Disabled People and Carers in Waltham Forest*, Waltham Forest Race Relations Unit, London

Berthoud, R., Lakey, J. and McKay, S. (1993) *The Economic Problems of Disabled People*, Policy Studies Institute, London

Battye, L. (1966) The Chatterly syndrome. In *Stigma: The Experience of Disability*, (ed. P. Hunt), Geoffrey Chapman, London

Biklen, D. and Bogdana, R. (1977) *Media Portrayal of Disabled People: A Study of Stereotypes*, Inter-Racial Children's Book Bulletin, **8**, **6** and **7**, 4–9

Broadcasting Standards Council (1989) *Annual Report 1988–89 and Code of Practice*, Broadcasting Standards Council, London

Cumberbatch, G., and Negrine, R. (1992) *Images of Disability on Television*, Routlege, London

Finkelstein, V. (1980) *Attitudes and Disabled People*, World Health Organization, Geneva

French, S. (1989) Mind your language. *Nursing Times*, **85**, **2**, 29–31

Gartner, A. and Joe, T. (1987) *Images of the Disabled; Disabling Images*, Preager, New York

Hevey, D. (1992) *The Creatures Time Forgot: Photography and Disability Imagery*, Routlege, London

HMSO (1991) *Social Trends 21*, Her Majesty's Stationary Office, London

Killin, D. (1993) Equal opportunities, disabled lesbians and disabled gay men and personal assistance in *Making Our Own Choices*, (ed. C. Barnes), Belper, British Council of Organisations of Disabled People

Lonsdale (1990) *Women and Disability*, Tavistock Macmillan, London

Martin, J. and White, A. (1988) *The Financial Circumstances of Disabled Adults Living in Private Households*, Her Majesty's Stationary Office, London

Morris, J. (1991) *Pride Against Prejudice*, The Women's Press, London

Oliver, M. (1990) *The Politics of Disablement*, Macmillan, Basingstoke

Reiser, R. (1992) Children's literature. In *Disability Equality in the Classroom: A Human Rights Issue*, (eds R. Reiser and M. Mason) Disability Equality in Education, London, 105–114

Smith, S. and Jordan, A. (1991) *What the Papers Say and Don't Say About Disability*, The Spastics Society, London

Sutherland, A. (1981) *Disabled We Stand*, Souvenir Press, London

Wertheimer, A. (1988) *According to the Papers: Press Reporting on People with Learning Difficulties*, Values Into Action, London

Without Walls (1991) *Selling Murder: The Killing Films of the Third Reich*, Domino Films, shown on Channel 4 on 22 October 1991

4

The disabled role

Sally French

Role is a sociological concept not a medical concept. Abercrombie et al. define roles as 'bundles of socially defined attributes and expectations associated with social positions' (1988: 209). All our roles contain certain rights and obligations. The student, for example, has the right to receive a good standard of education but is obliged to hand in essays on time and prepare for examinations; the employee has the right to work in a safe environment but is obliged to be punctual and to follow the instructions of supervisors. Most people occupy multiple roles: for example mother, employee, neighbour, daughter and friend. The person defined as ill occupies the 'sick role', and the person who becomes a patient occupies the 'patient role'.

Parsons (1951) was the first sociologist to elaborate the concept of the 'sick role'. He believed this role to contain two major rights and two major obligations:

Right One
The sick person is not responsible for his or her illness.

Right Two
The sick person is relieved of normal social responsibilities.

Obligation One
The sick person must view his or her condition as undesirable.

Obligation Two
The sick person must seek and co-operate with competent medical help.

Parsons thought that the second right, to be relieved of normal social responsibilities, was potentially desirable, and that, as this threatens social order, entry to the sick role must be controlled. The sick role legitimates illness, but it also regulates it so that social obligations are not evaded unnecessarily. Hart explains:

> If outbreaks of sickness were left to the whims of individuals in the private sphere of domestic life, they might gradually erode people's sense of duty to work, to family life, to community. Only by bringing sickness into the public sphere and encasing it in a system of social control would the risks of role evasion be kept to a minimum. (1985: 97)

People who occupy the sick role, yet appear to enjoy it and fail to seek medical help, are not keeping to their side of the bargain and are likely to meet with great disapproval from friends, family, employers and health and welfare professionals. Davis (1993) believes that disabled people are expected to play the sick role whether they are ill or not. Viewing disability and sickness as the same thing can be very detrimental to disabled people who are often extremely fit and healthy.

The 'sick role' model fits acute illness best. People with physical impairments or psychiatric illnesses may not be allowed to terminate their usual social duties, or may never be permitted to resume them (Scambler, 1982). Sutherland (1981) believes that disabled people are expected to accept and adjust to the limitations imposed upon them, to overcome the difficulties they face, and to be as independent and as 'normal' as possible. This, he considers, constitutes 'the disabled role'.

Characteristics of the disabled role

Independence

Physical independence, such as cooking, washing and dressing, is generally considered to be something disabled people desire above all else. In many ways this is so, for if a person is excessively dependent on others, then he or she must fit in with their schedules and plans with a subsequent loss of freedom and autonomy. In addition it is all too easy for the relationship to develop into an unequal one, with the helper having undue power and the disabled person being compelled constantly to express gratitude, or at best never to complain. This oppression is difficult to challenge because many disabled people need some assistance and its continuance may depend on expressing a sufficient degree of appreciation. As a disabled woman featured in Sutherland's book puts it, 'If you stand up for your rights you are biting the hand that feeds you and you will lose the support that you actually physically need to survive' (1981: 72).

Health and welfare professionals usually regard physical independence as a central aim in the rehabilitation process. Stewart, for example, states:

> It may not be easy for a nurse to stand back and watch an old lady struggling to get into her stockings while one hand lies helpless by her side, paralysed by a disabling stroke. Yet nurses who are rehabilitation orientated know that the patient must struggle towards independence. Any short-circuiting of the process will prolong the period of dependency. (1985: 14)

But is it always in the best interests of disabled people to strive for independence of this type? A disabled woman featured in Campling's book thinks not, she explains, 'I can sew but so slowly that it bores me to do it,' (1981: 1). Similarly, a person with a physical impairment may ask for assistance in cleaning, cooking and dressing, as so many non-disabled people do, in order to save time and energy to lead a full and satisfying life. Morris (1989) found that many of the women with spinal-cord injuries she interviewed chose to rely on personal assistance so that they could concentrate on other things, such as community work or political activity. Disabled people define independence, not in physical terms, but in terms of control. People who are almost totally dependent on others, in a physical sense, can still have independence of thought and action, enabling them to take full and active charge of their lives.

Impairments tend to make disabled people slow, which is inconvenient enough without making matters worse in a futile attempt to be independent. Narrowly defined, independence can give rise to inefficiency and stress, as well as wasting precious time. Technology, for example, may enable disabled people to perform a task unaided, but in a slow and inefficient way; Wolff (1986) points out that the excessive use of technology, in place of human help, can also give rise to social isolation. The pressures placed upon disabled people to achieve physical independence are regarded by Sutherland (1981) and Shearer (1981) as a form of oppression. Sutherland quotes a disabled person as saying:

> I've known a few people who, as adults, have refused to walk even though they could because its just not worth the effort. And people have often got angry with them, often. They've been labelled lazy and all sorts of things. They're definitely considered odd if they choose to be in a wheelchair, in the same way as you're considered odd if you don't struggle to do something that you can actually do even though it takes you six hours. (1981: 69)

Corbett (1989) agrees, believing that self-help skills can be an intolerable chore for some disabled people, impeding their quality of life and inhibiting self-expression. She describes how people with severe learning difficulties can actually regress if independence is forced upon them indiscriminately.

We are, of course, all dependent on each other to a large extent, and we all use aids, such as washing machines, scissors, motor cars, aeroplanes, eating utensils and computers, to save time and to overcome physical limitations such as our inability to move fast or to fly. We are also dependent on other people to produce and repair these aids. As Oliver points out, the dependency of disabled people 'is not a feature that marks them out as different in kind from the rest of the population but as different in degree' (1993: 51). Despite the inter-dependency of us all, the dependency of disabled people tends to be regarded as special, as qualitatively different.

The problems disabled people face and the equipment they need, such as wheelchairs and hoists, are also regarded as exceptional. This creates beliefs among health professionals and others that disabled people should 'manage' in as 'normal' a way as possible and that 'unnecessary' aids may harm them by reducing the amount of exercise they take or by making them lazy and dependent. These beliefs, and the control of professionals over resources, exacerbate the considerable practical difficulties disabled people face in acquiring the aids and equipment they need (Davis, 1993).

The physical and psychological stress involved in gaining independence in basic tasks, as well as the wasted time and reduced social opportunities incurred, are rarely given much attention by anyone other than disabled people themselves. Yet we do not insist that people walk six miles, or even one, rather than using their motor cars, or that they dispense with labour-saving devices in case they become lazy or dependent on the people who produced them. Indeed, to attempt to enforce such a plan would be considered extremely patronizing and a serious breach of human rights, even if it were motivated in terms of the person's 'own good'. Why then should people with motor impairments be denied electric wheelchairs just because they can physically manage to walk or push a manual one? Clearly disabled people are not enjoying the same freedom of choice as other citizens and are placed in an oppressive relationship with those who have control of their lives.

It is frequently the case that non-disabled people are dependent on disabled people in some way, perhaps as those with time to help or listen or, in the case of health and welfare professionals, as a way of earning their living! There is a huge commercial industry around disability providing lucrative work for many people (Greater Manchester Coalition of Disabled People, undated). A disabled person may also serve the needs, often incidentally, of those who want to care, be useful, or to help. There is often an erroneous assumption that disabled people are unable to reciprocate the help which they receive, whereas in reality people who require assistance are often carers themselves (Potts and Fido, 1991; Morris, 1991; Parker, 1993; Walmsley, 1993). Brechin and Swain argue that 'dependence on others is a vital aspect of personal development and an essential and *continuing* component of personal autonomy' (1982: 58).

Paradoxically, although disabled people are often under enormous pressure to be 'independent', Oliver (1993) argues that other pressures—economic, political and professional—operate to maintain disabled people in a dependent and helpless state. Sutherland (1981) believes that disabled people are expected to play the 'weak and needy' role, receiving help with gratitude even when it is not needed; charities are prime examples of large organizations which have depicted disabled people in this way (see chapter 3). Disabled people are frequently socialized into a dependent role which makes it very difficult for them to take control of their lives if and when the opportunity to do so arises. As Sutherland puts it, 'people are conditioned to play roles which serve the needs of their oppressors' (1981: 71).

This confusion between dependence and independence can best be understood by focusing on the needs of the non-disabled community. In many ways it is in the interests of society, with regard to both convenience and cost, for disabled people to achieve independence in daily living tasks. On the other hand, it may be convenient for society to maintain disabled people in a dependent state, as their independence may require expensive change, such as the building of a barrier-free environment. As mentioned above, a large number of people also rely on the dependency of disabled people to earn their living (Davis, 1993).

Normality

Closely associated with the concept of independence is that of normality. The pressures placed upon disabled people to appear 'normal' can give rise to enormous inefficiency and stress, yet many disabled people are well into adulthood before they realize what is happening or before they find the courage to abandon such attempts (Campling, 1981). Sutherland talks at length of this, believing that:

> We are subjected to continual pressure to conform to a 'normal' image, this is one of the major reasons for the manufacture of elaborate prosthetic limbs and hands, which are often poor substitutes for the purely functional devices such as wooden legs or metal hooks which they replace. (1981: 75)

The pressure to be 'normal' is often at the expense of the disabled person's needs and rights. For example, if a person with a motor impairment who can walk short distances is denied a wheelchair, he or she may become isolated or unsuitable for certain types of education or employment. Mason believes that, 'almost every activity of daily living can take on the dimension of trying to make you less like yourself and more like the able-bodied' (1992: 27), and Ryan and Thomas (1987) contend that the conventional and conformist life styles forced upon disabled people can be an exaggeration of normality. Munro and Elder-Woodward state:

> Service users should not *have* to conform to the standards and values of the majority of society, nor to the expectations of service providers, they should have access to the full range of possibilities so that they can make choices using their own values and interests (1992: 29)

The goal of 'normality' can also be physically dangerous, as when the person with a serious visual impairment avoids using a white stick. In addition, rendering an impairment less visible can create social problems which are equally or more difficult to manage than when the impairment is exposed. As a disabled woman in Sutherland's book explains, 'I'm happier with something that isn't a deception than with something that is' (1981: 75). Sutherland, drawing heavily on the experiences of disabled people in encounters with health professionals, talks at length of this. He states:

> There's a tremendous emphasis on a child who's had polio or whatever to walk, to be as able-bodied as possible. It's like standing up is infinitely better than sitting down, even if you're standing up in a total frame—metal straps and God knows what—that weighs a ton, that you can't move in, which hurts, takes hours to get on and off and looks ugly. It's assumed that that's what you want and that's what is best for you. (1981: 72)

Many disabled people are well into adulthood before they manage to abandon, or at least challenge, these expectations of 'normality'. For most this is a gradual process which comes with the confidence of age, but for some it can be a sudden realization. A deaf woman in Campling's book had such an experience when she saw a group of deaf people in a restaurant, she states: 'They were laughing and talking and didn't give a damn that the whole place knew they were deaf. . . . My years of pretence seemed suddenly absurd. I had been making life "normal" and easy for everyone except myself' (1981: 36).

Therapists and nurses may also believe that the ways in which disabled people move and communicate are inferior to those of non-disabled people, a notion which many disabled people, especially those from the deaf community, have hotly disputed. The concept of 'normality' is often accepted uncritically. In Tarver et al., three therapists, state:

> Being in a wheelchair may give you mobility but it is a highly abnormal form of mobility with all kinds of disadvantages—practical and social. Communication through gesture or writing, or a communication aid is not normal human communication. It may be the only way to get your message across but it is still comparatively inefficient and open to misunderstanding (1993: 7)

Because of the negative attitudes towards disability which prevail in society, disabled people and those who live and work with them, may come to the conclusion that attempting to be 'normal' is the only way to succeed; the goal of normality is thus justified in terms of social acceptance. For example, it can be argued that one of the objectives of deaf people learning to talk, blind people learning to use facial expression appropriately and people with Down's syndrome having plastic surgery, is that they will be more socially acceptable, less isolated and better able to compete with non-disabled people. Although these ideas contain some truth, the problem with this approach is that disabled people must carry the entire burden of disability themselves, while society learns nothing of its true nature. These expectations lead many disabled people to try and become 'superhuman' so as to avoid the negative stereotypes of helplessness and inadequacy. Morris (1991) contends that those who play the role of 'honorary non-disabled person' do little to further the interests of disabled people as a whole. This type of behaviour is, however, often rewarded by professionals and encouraged in the professional literature (Swaffield, 1986).

Morris (1993a) believes that the assumption that disabled people want to be normal, rather than just as they are, is one of the most oppressive experiences to which they are subjected. She rejects the view that it is progressive and liberating to ignore difference, believing that disabled people have a right to be both equal and different. She states 'I do not want to have to try to emulate what a non-disabled woman looks like in order to assert positive things about myself. I want to be able to celebrate my difference, not hide from it,' (Morris, 1991: 184). Abberley points out that any abnormality which disabled people demonstrate results not from their impairments but 'from the failure of society to meet our "normal" needs as impaired people' (1993: 111).

The emphasis on normality can also lead non-disabled people to deny or fail to believe that a person's impairment or disability exists, particularly with those with relatively hidden impairments who manage to 'pass' as normal. This gives rise to the erroneous assumption that disabled people are 'just like everyone else' a notion which is advocated by Fenton (1992), and by the Royal National Institute for the Blind who state 'The biggest compliment you can pay a visually impaired person is to forget that she has impaired vision' (RNIB Factsheet, undated: 9). This lack of acceptance by non-disabled people of the reality of disability, can lead disabled people to deny and minimize the oppression and difficulties they face. Talking of childhood French explains:

> I denied my disability in response to their denial which was often motivated by a benign attempt to integrate me in a world which they perceived as fixed. My denial of disability was thus not a psychopathological reaction, but a sensible and rational response to the peculiar situation I was in. (1993: 70)

Similarly Morris states:

> our anger is not about having 'a chip on your shoulder', our grief is not 'a failure to come to terms with disability'. Our dissatisfaction with our lives is not a personality defect but a sane response to the oppression we experience. (1993b: 67)

Sutherland believes that disabled people are pressurized into accepting their situation by being told that it does not exist, and Hevey, talking of people with hidden disabilities, states:

> We are constructed as refugees at the border between disability and non-disability. The guards survey us and issue passports into the promised land if we agree to internalise our oppression or pretend that it doesn't exist. Many people with hidden impairments feel close enough to the promised (non-disabled) land to attempt to 'pass'. (1992: 81)

Acceptance and adjustment

Therapists, nurses and others have viewed their role as one of helping disabled people 'accept' their disabilities and 'adjust' to them. Talking of visually impaired people, Stewart states 'acceptance must precede rehabilitation' and that 'if acceptance must precede rehabilitation, it follows that non-acceptance will obstruct rehabilitation' (1985: 194). Disabled people have been urged to 'overcome' what are viewed as 'their' problems, to learn to live with them and never to complain. Any anger or depression concerning lack of access, negative attitudes, inappropriate rehabilitation, poor housing, or non-existent educational or job prospects, have been viewed as evidence of maladjustment, denial, and 'chips on their shoulders'.

As well as making a physical adjustment it is assumed that the disabled person must also make a psychological adjustment. It is thought that becoming disabled is inevitably psychologically devastating, a personal tragedy. Carroll (1961) likened the loss of sight to dying, and many people, for example Weller and Miller (1977), believe that the adjustment to disability requires a process of mourning. There has certainly been a growing trend towards counselling by health and welfare professionals indicating a developing psychological orientation. Oliver (1983), however, rejects such ideas on the grounds that non-disabled people view disability and adjustment in terms of the individual, thus neglecting wider social influences. He has also found that these explanations fail to tally with the experiences of many disabled people who neither grieve nor mourn and who may indeed find the experience of disability enriching. Even people who do mourn may be mourning the loss of their independence rather than the loss of bodily function or appearance, a situation which could to a large extent be eliminated by social and environmental change.

Finkelstein (1981) speculates that grief models have arisen as non-disabled professionals have tried to imagine what it is like to be disabled. Although some people may find the onset of impairment devastating, the psychological state of disabled people appears to reflect that of the population generally. It is also the experience of many disabled people that becoming disabled opens up new and satisfying opportunities (British Psychological Society, 1989).

Scott (1969) found that professionals working with visually-impaired people tended to regard their clients' problems in psychological terms. This was in contrast to the visually-impaired people themselves who viewed the difficulties arising from their blindness as practical problems. Scott noted that the difficulties expressed by the visually-impaired people were often referred to by the professionals as 'the presenting problem', implying superficiality. He states:

> Workers regard the client's initial definition of his problems as akin to the visible portion of an iceberg. Beneath the surface of awareness lies a tremendously complicated mass of problems that must be dealt with before the surface problems can ever be solved. (1969: 77)

Oliver (1983) believes that these psychological theories may become self-fulfilling, with the disabled person concluding that disability is tragic and behaving accordingly. Treischmann (1980) points out that disabled people cannot win, for if they show no evidence of a psychological reaction following the onset of disability they are assumed to be demonstrating denial which is in itself viewed as a psychological problem.

The notion that disabled people should accept their situation and adjust to it thus arises from individualistic models of disability, where it is conceptualized as a relatively unchangeable, internal state, rather than the result of physical and social barriers which could be removed if the political will to do so was there. Individualistic conceptions of disability have been severely criticized by disabled people who have concluded that they serve the interests, not of themselves, but of the non-disabled majority. It is very convenient for society that disabled people should accept what are viewed as *their* problems and adjust to them, for in that way the status quo is maintained.

Disabled children have been socialized from an early age into believing that the rights of non-disabled people do not apply to them: it is often those who become disabled later in life who see most clearly that by accepting disability and adjusting to it, they are, in effect, relinquishing their citizenship rights. As Sutherland states:

> People who acquire their disabilities in adult life are in a very different position. They have much more power than children . . . which makes it easier for them to reject attempts to stereotype them or make them

conform to a role they find undesirable. Having had the opportunity to establish a place in the world and become secure in their individual identity they are also more likely to recognise such attempts clearly for what they are and to have the confidence to contradict them. (1981: 95)

Taking responsibility

As well as the expectation that disabled people should accept and adjust to their situation, they are also expected to take full responsibility for the feelings non-disabled people have about impairment and disability, and to cope with any problems which arise in social interaction. In order to achieve this, disabled people are forced to behave in ways which are often detrimental to themselves; people with epilepsy may, for example, be expected to explain constantly their condition and offer reassurance, deaf people may struggle to lip read, and visually-impaired people may endure boredom rather than 'spoiling other people's fun'. Having to take responsibility in this way also prevents disabled people from sharing their experiences and anxieties.

In contrast, non-disabled people are not expected to understand deafness, blindness, epilepsy or paralysis, or to alter their behaviour in any substantial way. If they do make any concessions disabled people are expected to show gratitude even though they are required, as a matter of course, to adjust their behaviour most of the time. The feeling that favours are being granted can make disabled people apologetic (for their very existence) as well as inhibiting them from demanding what they need. Sutherland (1981) makes the point that non-disabled people frequently get angry if disabled people so much as mention their oppression.

Internal oppression

We are oppressed from without by a society which does not value us and therefore does not give priority to our needs, and we are oppressed from within because we have internalised these same attitudes towards ourselves. (Woolley 1993: 81)

As well as the external oppression disabled people experience from other people's attitudes and expectations, disabled people can also become internally oppressed by viewing themselves in the same way as non-disabled people view them, and behaving as others expect them to behave. This self-fulfilling prophecy can, in turn, lead to 'proof' that the erroneous attitudes and beliefs about disabled people are correct, which can serve to justify the treatment they receive, creating a vicious circle (Finkelstein and French, 1993: 32). Wolfenberger and Tullman contend that 'The social roles that people impose on each other or adopt are among the most powerful social influences and control methods known' (1989: 215). Despite this, it is not unusual for disabled people to merely *comply* with the roles imposed on them, for example, until their rehabilitation is complete.

It is not at all surprising that disabled people internalize the views of the wider society as, with the exception of the indigenous deaf community, there has been very little sense of cultural identity among them until recent times. This makes it difficult for disabled people to reject the expectations and beliefs about how they should think and behave, which non-disabled people hold. Disabled children, in particular, are very vulnerable to this conditioning. Their parents are often unwitting oppressors in the process, with their beliefs and expectations being shaped by those of professional 'experts' and society at large. In this way the disabled role can become part of the disabled person's sense of self and identity. As Morris states:

> Most of the people we have dealings with, including our most intimate relationships, are not like us. It is therefore very difficult for us to recognise and challenge the values and judgements that are applied to us and our lives. Our ideas about disability and about ourselves are generally formed by those who are not disabled. (1991: 37)

The disabled role is rarely completely internalized, however, not least because of its contradictory nature. Nevertheless, most disabled people spend a great deal of time and energy both playing the role and attempting to reverse their conditioning. The growing cultural identity of disabled people, and the disability movement, have put forward new and radical interpretations of disability which offer disabled people affirmation and support as they redefine their situation. (For further information on the disability movement, the reader is referred to chapter 6.)

Denial

If disabled people dare to challenge the stereotypes people have of them, or refuse to play the disabled role, they are likely to be confronted with unpleasant reactions. To protect themselves from this, disabled people learn from their earliest childhood to deny or minimize their disabilities. This process has been analysed in detail by French (1993) who concludes that disabled people deny their experience of disability for the following reasons:

- To avoid other people's anxiety and distress.
- To avoid other people's disappointment and frustration.

- To avoid other people's disbelief.
- To avoid other people's rejection.
- To avoid other people's disapproval.
- To live up to other people's ideas of 'normality'.
- To avoid spoiling other people's fun.
- To collude with other people's pretences.

French believes that disabled people deny their reality of disability, not because of flaws in their individual psyches, but for social, economic and emotional survival, and that they do so at considerable cost to their sense of self and their identities. She contends, 'When people deny our disabilities they deny who we really are' (1993: 74).

Conclusion

Disabled people are conditioned from their earliest childhood to *manage* and *overcome* disability, to be independent, to be 'normal' and to play the disabled role. This has led to a dearth of information on the real experience of disability, as well as a lack of debate on the best ways of improving the lives of disabled people.

Nurses and therapists have considerable power over disabled people and have played their part, often unwittingly, in imposing the disabled role upon them. Disabled people are now organizing themselves to fight the oppression they face. If nurses and therapists are to maintain the respect of disabled people they must widen and deepen their knowledge of disability and join disabled people in their fight for justice.

Finkelstein (1991) argues that once a 'cure or care' interpretation of disability is abandoned, all sorts of exciting possibilities become apparent. This is not to imply that helping a disabled person to gain physical independence, or psychological acceptance, is inappropriate, but to stress the importance of health and welfare professionals understanding the social construction of disability and the processes by which disabled people are compelled to play a role which not only fails to meet their needs, but renders them second-class beings.

References

Abberley, P. (1993) Disabled people and normality. In *Disabling Barriers—Enabling Environments*, (eds J. Swain, V. Finkelstein, S. French and M. Oliver), Sage, London

Abercrombie, N., Hill, S. and Turner, B. (1988) *Dictionary of Sociology*, Penguin Books, Harmondsworth

Brechin, A. and Swain, J. (1982) Mental handicap and integration. Unit 8 of the Open University Course *The Handicapped Person in the Community*, The Open University, Milton Keynes

British Psychological Society (1989) *Psychology and Physical Disability in the National Health Service* Report of the Professional Affaires Board of The British Psychological Society, Leicester

Campling, J. (ed.) (1981) *Images of Ourselves: Women with Disabilities Talking*, Routledge & Kegan Paul, London

Carroll, T. J. (1961) Blindness—what it is, what it does and how to live with it. Cited in *Social Work and Disabled People*, (1983) (M. Oliver), Macmillan, London

Corbett, J. (1989) The quality of life in the 'independence' curriculum. *Disability, Handicap and Society*, **4 (2)**, 145–163

Davis, K. (1993) The crafting of good clients. In *Disabling Barriers—Enabling Environments*, (eds J. Swain, V. Finkelstein, S. French and M. Oliver), Sage, London

Fenton, M. (1992) *Working Together Towards Independence*, The Royal Association for Disability and Rehabilitation, London

Finkelstein, V. (1981) Disability and the helper/helped relationship: an historical view. In *Handicap in a Social World*, (eds A. Brechin, P. Liddiard and J. Swain), Hodder & Stoughton, Sevenoaks

Finkelstein, V. (1991) Disability: an administrative challenge. In *Social Work, Disabled People and Disabling Environments*, (ed. M. Oliver), Jessica Kingsley, London

Finkelstein, V. and French, S. (1993) Towards a psychology of disability. In *Disabling Barriers—Enabling Environments*, (eds J. Swain, V. Finkelstein, S. French and M. Oliver), Sage, London

French, S. (1993) 'Can you see the rainbow?' the roots of denial. In *Disabling Barriers—Enabling Environments*, (eds J. Swain, V. Finkelstein, S. French and M. Oliver), Sage, London

Greater Manchester Coalition of Disabled People (undated) *Making Money Out of Disability*, GMCDP, Manchester

Hart, N. (1985) *The Sociology of Health and Medicine*, Causeway Press, Ormskirk.

Hevey, D. (1992) *The Creatures Time Forgot: Photography and Disability Imagery*, Routledge, London

Mason, M. (1992) Internalised oppression. In *Disability Equality in the Classroom: A Human Rights Issue*, (2nd ed), (eds R. Rieser and M. Mason) Disability Equality in Education, London

Morris, J. (1989) *Able Lives*, The Women's Press, London

Morris, J. (1991) *Pride Against Prejudice*, The Women's Press, London

Morris, J. (1993a) Prejudice. In *Disabling Barriers—Enabling Environments*, (eds J. Swain, V. Finkelstein, S. French and M. Oliver), Sage, London

Morris, J. (1993b) Feminism and disability. *Feminist Review*, Spring, **43**, 57–70

Munro, K. and Elder-Woodward, J. (1992) *Independent Living*, Churchill Livingstone, Edinburgh

Oliver, M. (1983) *Social Work and Disabled People*, Macmillan, London

Oliver, M. (1993) Disability and dependency: a creation of industrial societies? In *Disabling Barriers—Enabling Environments*, (eds J. Swain, V. Finkelstein, S. French and M. Oliver), Sage, London

Parker, G. (1993) *With this Body: Caring and Disability in Marriage*, Open University Press, Buckingham

Parsons, T. (1951) *The Social System*, Routledge & Kegan Paul, London

Potts, M. and Fido, R. (1991) *'A Fit Person to be Removed' Personal Accounts of Life in a Mental Deficiency Institution*, Northcote House, Plymouth

RNIB Factsheet (undated) *A Short Guide to Blindness*, Royal National Institute for the Blind, London

Ryan, J. and Thomas, F. (1987) *The Politics of Mental Handicap* Free Association Books, London

Scambler, G. (1982) Illness behaviour. In *Sociology as Applied to Medicine*, (eds D. L. Patrick and G. Scambler), Bailliere Tindall, London

Scott, R. A. (1969) *The Making of Blind Men*, Russell Sage Foundation, New York

Shearer, A. (1981) *Disability: Whose Handicap?* Basil Blackwell, Oxford

Stewart, W. (1985) *Counselling in Rehabilitation*, Croom Helm, London

Sutherland, A. T. (1981) *Disabled We Stand*, Souvenir Press, London

Swaffield, L. (1986) Every day a miracle. *Therapy Weekly*, **13 (17)**, 4

Tarver, M. A., Benson, S. and Thomas, G. (1993) Therapists' approaches to the emotional needs of their patients. Paper presented at the Mental Health Needs of Disabled People conference, 3rd March, Douglas Bader Centre, Queen Mary's University Hospital, Roehampton

Treischmann, R. B. (1980) *Spinal Cord Injuries*, Pergamon Press, Oxford

Walmsley, J. (1993) Contradictions in caring: reciprocity and interdependence. *Disability, Handicap and Society*, **8 (2)**, 129–141

Weller, D. J. and Miller, P. M. (1977) Emotional reactions of patient, family and staff in the acute care period of spinal cord injury. Cited in *Social Work and Disabled People*, (1983) (M. Oliver), Macmillan, London

Wolfenberger, W. and Tullman, S. (1989) A brief outline of the principle of normalisation. In *Making Connections*, (A. Brechin and J. Walmsley), Hodder & Stoughton, London

Wolff, H. (1986) The disabled student in 2001—deserted or liberated by new technology? *Educare*, **24**, 3–8

Woolley, M. (1993) Acquired hearing loss: acquired oppression. In *Disabling Barriers—Enabling Environments*, (eds J. Swain, V. Finkelstein, S. French and M. Oliver), Sage, London

5

Prejudice

Jenny Morris

Since becoming disabled, I have on countless occasions been told by both strangers and acquaintances how 'wonderful' they think I am. I eventually realized that at the heart of such remarks lay the judgement that being disabled must be awful, indeed intolerable. It is very undermining to realize that people look at me and see an experience which they would do everything to avoid for themselves.

How can we take pride in ourselves when disability provokes such negative feelings among non-disabled people? In answering this question disabled people have developed an understanding of the nature of prejudice and its effect on us.

Normality, difference and prejudice

Prejudice is associated with the recognition of difference. In theory 'normal' could be a value-free word to mean merely that which is common, and to be different from normal would not therefore necessarily provoke prejudice. In practice, the word is inherently tied up with ideas about what is right, what is desirable and what belongs.

Disabled people are not normal in the eyes of non-disabled people. Our physical and intellectual characteristics are not 'right' or 'admirable' and we do not 'belong'. Having given such a negative meaning to abnormality, the non-disabled world assumes that we wish to be normal or to be treated as if we were. It is supposedly progressive and liberating to ignore our differences because these differences have such negative meanings for non-disabled people. But we *are* different. We reject the meanings that the non-disabled world attaches to disability but we do not reject the differences which are such an important part of our identities.

Prejudice lies at the heart of the segregation which many disabled people experience both as children and as adults—and has its most extreme expression in the mass slaughter of disabled people under the German Third Reich. Prejudice can, however, also take more subtle forms. Hidden assumptions form the bedrock to most of our interaction with the non-disabled world. It is often difficult for us to identify *why* someone's behaviour makes us angry, or feel undermined. Our anger and insecurity can thus seem unreasonable not just to others but also, sometimes to ourselves.

From her interaction with non-disabled people, Pam Evans has identified a number of assumptions which are held about disabled people:

That we feel ugly, inadequate and ashamed of our disability.

That our lives are a burden to us, barely worth living.

That we crave to be 'normal' and 'whole'.

That whatever we choose to do or think, any work or pursuit we undertake is done as 'therapy', with the sole intention of taking our mind off our condition.

That we don't have, and never have had, any real or significant experiences in the way that non-disabled people do.

That we can't ever really accept our condition, and if we appear to be leading a full and contented life, or are simply cheerful, we are just 'putting a brave face on it.'

That we need 'taking out of ourselves' with diversions and rewards that only the normal world can provide.

That we desire to emulate and achieve normal behaviour and appearance in all things.

That we go about the daily necessities or pursue an interest because it is a 'challenge' through which we can 'prove' ourselves capable.

That we feel envy and resentment of the able-bodied.

That any emotion or distress we show can only be due to our disability and not to the same things that hurt and upset them.

That our disability has affected us psychologically, making us bitter and neurotic.

That it's quite amazing if we laugh, are cheerful and pleasant or show pleasure in other people's happiness.

That we are ashamed of our inabilities, our 'abnormalities', and loathe our wheelchairs, crutches or other aids.

That we never 'give up hope' of a cure.

That the inability to walk, to see or to hear is infinitely more dreadful than any other physical aspect of disability.

That words like 'walk' and 'dance' will upset us.

That when we affirm that we cannot, or do not wish to do something, our judgement and preferences are overridden and contradicted as inferior to theirs.

That we are asexual or at best sexually inadequate.

That if we are not married or in a long-term relationship it is because no one wants us and not through any personal choice to remain single or to live alone.

That any able-bodied person who marries us must have done so for one of the following suspicious motives and *never* through love: desire to hide his/her own inadequacies in the disabled person's obvious ones; an altruistic and saintly desire to sacrifice their lives to our care; neurosis of some sort; or plain old-fashioned fortune-hunting.

That if we have a partner who is also disabled, we chose each other for no other reason and not for any other qualities we might possess. When we choose 'our own kind' in this way the able-bodied world feels relieved, until of course we wish to have children; then we're seen as irresponsible.

That if our marriage or relationship fails, it is entirely due to our disability and the difficult person this inevitably makes us, and never from the usual things that make any relationship fail.

That those of us whose disability is such that we require a carer to attend to our physical needs are helpless cabbages who don't do anything and have nothing to give, and who lead meaningless, empty lives.

That if we are particularly gifted, successful or attractive before the onset of disability, our fate is infinitely more 'tragic' than if we were none of these things.

That we should put up with any inconvenience, discomfort or indignity in order to participate in 'normal' activities and events. And that this will somehow 'do us good'.

That our need of and right to privacy isn't as important as theirs, and that our lives need to be monitored in a way that deprives us of privacy and choice.

(Pam Evans, from an interview with the author.)

We could also add the assumption that disabled people could not possibly be lesbians or gay, and that if we are this is because we cannot achieve a 'normal' heterosexual relationship rather than being an expression of our sexuality. Nasa Begum drew my attention to some of the assumptions imposed on black and ethnic minority disabled people. These include the assumption that, as she put it, 'it is our ethnic culture that restricts our lives as disabled people' and that 'we should be grateful for the services we receive in Western societies, because we wouldn't be able to get them in our own countries.'

One of the biggest problems for disabled people is that all these undermining messages become part of our way of thinking about ourselves and/or our thinking about other disabled people. This is the internalization of *their* values about *our* lives.

Although overt hostility is not a common experience for most disabled people, it is yet the iron fist in the velvet glove of the patronizing and seemingly benevolent attitudes which we experience. This is clear from the experience of those of us who step out from the passive role which society accords to us. In these situations we often have to confront dislike, revulsion and fear.

The importance of physical difference

In an interview with me, Molly McIntosh talked of other people's reactions to physical difference.

> I have horrible scars on my face. What I mean by that is that people react to them with horror. Forty years ago when I was in my twenties, and also when I was a child, I so hated the way that I looked I tried not to think about it but every time I went out in the street I would be reminded about how I looked because of the way people reacted to me. As I walked down the street and someone was coming towards me, they would look and then drop their eyes or move their head, as if the horror was too much. But then they could never, ever resist looking again.

Molly McIntosh felt that her life was split in two. When she was at home she felt at ease with herself but when she set foot outside her front door she felt a deep sense of unease. Most of us experience the same sense of unease each time we interact with the non-disabled world, particularly in a public situation where we are dealing with strangers' reactions to us.

Going out in public so often takes courage. How many of us find that we can't dredge up the strength to do it day after day, week after week, year after year, a lifetime of rejection and revulsion? It is not only physical limitations which restrict us to our homes and those whom we know, it is the knowledge that each entry into the public world will be dominated by stares, by condescension, by pity and by hostility.

Some of us find that the only way we can survive in a non-disabled world is either not to recognize how much we are feared and hated, or to pretend that we don't know about it. Some of us feel that we can confront the stares and hostility head on. I talked to Anna Mathison, who lives in a black community in which she feels she belongs. She has the confidence to refuse to be intimidated by other people's reactions to her: 'If people stare I shout "What are you staring at? You want to feel? You need glasses?" I feel I should challenge them because otherwise they think you're stupid and that they are entitled to stare.'

However, Anna remains all too aware that people look at her and think her life is not worth living. 'They just see the wheelchair and they think, you'd be better off dead. And that's a problem because it hurts. But if I shout at them it makes me strong.'

We receive so many messages from the non-disabled world that we are not wanted, that we are considered less than human. For those with restricted mobility or sensory impairments, the very physical environment tells us we don't belong. It tells us that we aren't wanted in the places that non-disabled people spend their lives—their homes, their schools and colleges, their workplaces, their leisure venues. The refusal to give British Sign Language the status of a language means that deaf people are forced to use a language suited to people with different biological characteristics. The refusal to give Braille the same status as printed material shuts out people with a visual impairment. As Susan Hannaford writes, 'For no access read apartheid' (Hannaford 1985: 121).

Rachel Cartwright, who was born blind, talked to me about her experience of exclusion:

> All through my childhood, I felt set apart from my brothers and sisters. I went to a different school and because it was a residential school I felt as if I wasn't part of my family a lot of the time. When my parents thought about our future, they always thought in different terms when it came to me. As a child and as an adult I've been very aware of being excluded by the way that most printed material is not available on tape or in Braille, and that if it is it is only because a special favour has been made—for which I'm supposed to feel grateful.

Such exclusion gives us a clear message about the attitude of non-disabled people towards us.

Our physical or intellectual differences make us less than human in the eyes of non-disabled people, we can be excluded from normal human activity because we are not normally human. A physically different body, or a body which behaves in a different way, means an incomplete body and this means that our very selves are similarly incomplete.

Non-disabled people feel that our difference gives them the right to invade our privacy and make judgements about our lives. Our physical characteristics evoke such strong feelings that people often have to express them in some way. At the same time they feel able to impose their feelings on us because we are not considered to be autonomous human beings.

Many of us have experienced the total stranger or the slight acquaintance coming up and asking us the most intimate things about our lives. Our physical difference makes our bodies public property. Clare Robson experienced this when—as a result of having multiple sclerosis—one side of her body started shaking and she had to use a stick to help her to walk. 'People would come up to me in the street and ask me what was wrong. If I told them they would say "Oh how awful, there's no cure for that, is there?" '

Looking at someone with a physical disability does not always have the effect of undermining the disabled person. There is a difference between staring and gazing. As one young woman put it:

> Now some people can look at me for ever and I wouldn't care. Those are the people who seem to see, not just the best of me, but the most of me. They're not staring, they're gazing. A stare is kind of like a vampire bite—it sucks life out of you. A gaze is just the opposite—a love transfusion. (Disability Rights Education and Defence Fund 1982: 50)

Wanting to be normal

One of the most oppressive features of the prejudice which disabled people experience is the assumption that we want to be other than we are, that is we want to be normal. Yet, as Pam Evans says, 'Do we only have value, even to ourselves, in direct relation to how closely we can imitate "normal" appearance, function, belief and behaviour?' We may have the same aspirations as non-disabled people (in terms of how we live our lives) but quite patently we are not just like them in that we have physical differences which distinguish us from the majority of the population. Nevertheless the pressures on us to aspire to be 'normal' are huge – 'friends and family all conspire from the kindest and highest of intention to ensure we make the wrong choice', says Pam. 'Better to betray ourselves than them!'

I myself prefer to go shopping with my child because her presence at my side gives me, I mistakenly think, a passport into the world of normal people. To assert that I am a mother is to distance myself from the abnormality of being disabled. Some of us take pride in 'looking normal except for sitting down'. Very few of us feel able to celebrate our physical difference, although more of us do as the disability movement grows stronger.

One of the most important features of our experience of prejudice is that we generally experience it as isolated individuals. Many of us spend most of our lives in the company of non-disabled people, whether in our families, with friends, in the workplace, at school and so on. Most of the people we have dealings with, including in our most intimate relationships, are not like us. It is therefore very difficult for us to recognize and challenge the values and judgements that are applied to us and our lives. Our ideas about disability and about ourselves are generally formed by those who are not disabled.

In this situation, the emergence of a disability culture is difficult but tremendously liberating. Such a culture enables us to recognize the pressure to pretend to be normal for the oppressive and impossible-to-achieve hurdle which it is. More importantly, this culture challenges our own prejudices about ourselves, as well as those of the non-disabled culture. This is vital for, as Pam Evans says:

> Just as no feminist would think of trying to change discriminatory laws and conventions of society without *first* changing her own attitudes to her personal inheritance of conditioning, so no disabled person should see liberation from prejudice as solely a matter of changing others. The real liberation is essentially our own. For we are all accomplices to the prejudice in exact proportion to the values and norms of our society that we are prepared to endorse.

She goes on, 'We are *not* normal in the stunted terms the world chooses to define. But we are not obliged to adopt those definitions as standards to which we must aspire, or indeed, regard as something worth having in the first place.' Physical disability and illness are an important part of human experience. The non-disabled world may wish to try to ignore this and to react to physical difference by treating us as if we are not quite human, but we must recognize that our difference is both an essential part of human experience and, given the chance, can create important and different ways of looking at things.

References

Disability Rights Education and Defense Fund (1982) *No More Stares*, DREDF, Berkeley, CA

Hannaford, S. (1985) *Living Outside Inside* Canterbury Press, Berkeley, CA

(This paper is an edited version of a chapter that was originally published in J. Morris (1991) *Pride Against Prejudice: Transforming Attitudes towards Disability*, The Women's Press, London. It was published in its present form In *Disabling Barriers—Enabling Environments*, (eds J. Swain, V. Finkelstein, S. French and M. Oliver), Sage, London.)

6

The disability movement

Sally French

> Disabled people, like children, are meant to be seen and not heard, they are meant to be grateful not angry, they are meant to be humble not proud. In challenging all these preconceptions and discriminatory ideologies, the movement is making progress every day, even before attaining the central political objectives. (Shakespeare 1993: 262)

Social movements arise as a result of specific or widespread grievances; their goal is usually to reorganize society in some fundamental way (Abercrombie et al., 1988). Social movements have been defined by Giddens as 'a collective attempt to further a common interest, or secure a common goal, through collective action outside the sphere of established institutions' (1989: 624).

Disabled people, by virtue of their numbers, constitute, potentially, a powerful political force; yet because of the widespread discrimination against them, in terms of education, employment and access generally, disabled people are rendered relatively powerless. This lack of access and power applies as much to the political system as to any other area of life. It is extremely difficult for disabled people to become active participants in mainstream politics or to feed their ideas into the system. As Enticott et al. state:

> People with disabilities are excluded from the political system as they are in many other areas of life. Many are prevented from entering their local polling station and are offered an inadequate, discriminatory alternative; they are excluded from receiving wide ranging information on what they might vote for and why; their issues are treated as belonging to a minority—although they make up 14% of the electorate; they are excluded from believing they can change anything through politics and left feeling cynical and disillusioned. As a result they are prevented from playing their full and rightful part in society. (1992: 30)

The disability movement is a social movement which aims to empower disabled people by redefining disability from impairment and individual tragedy to social oppression, and by organizing society accordingly (Wood, 1990). Mason believes that the disability movement:

is not an organisation, although its power comes from disabled people's own organisations, but is rather a political analysis of the problem of disability. Any disabled person who has come to any part of the analysis and who tries to communicate that through language, policy or practice, is part of the disability movement. (1992a:16)

Oliver (1990) places the disability movement among the 'new social movements' which have emerged during the late twentieth century; the women's movement and the black people's movement are other examples. The aim of these movements is to gain equality, social justice, and participative democracy. New social movements take a critical stance to society, frequently crossing national boundaries. They are marginalized politically, but are almost always to the left of the political spectrum.

Driedger (1989) refers to the disability movement as 'the last civil rights movement'; it has certainly been influenced by the women's and black people's movements, and aspires to gain the rights which these groups have won, for example anti-discrimination legislation. The disability movement is not identical to these movements, however, for as Morris (1991) points out, although it is not inherently distressing to be a woman or to be black, it can be to be ill or in pain.

The disability movement in Great Britain has also been influenced by similar movements of disabled people abroad who, owing to the more favourable political climates in which they operate, have made greater progress. In the USA, for example, the civil rights movement became the vehicle for disabled activists (Pagel, 1988). This eventually led to the passing, in 1990, of the Americans with Disabilities Act which outlaws inaccessible buildings, inaccessible transport and discrimination in employment.

The history and growth of the disability movement

The movement came when disabled individuals first faced up to the fact that they could achieve more for themselves through collective action than they could on their own. (Davis, 1993: 287)

Organizations *of* disabled people are those where a substantial number of disabled people, 50 per cent or more, are in positions of control. Two early organizations of this type in Great Britain were the British Deaf Association (founded in 1890), which had its roots in the indigenous deaf community, and The National League of the Blind (founded in 1898). They were greatly influenced by the rise of the Trade Union and Labour movements. These early groups were militant, focusing on the particular problems deaf and blind people encounter when attempting to operate in a non-disabled world. In

1902 the National League of the Blind became affiliated to the Trade Union Congress and was the first trade union comprised of disabled people. It had many conflicts with charitable organizations believing them to have strong vested interest in maintaining blind people in their disadvantaged position (Pagel, 1988).

Over the next sixty years, many other organizations of disabled people developed. They usually focused on specific impairments or single issues, such as lack of State provision. These organizations clearly demonstrated the ability of disabled people to organize themselves democratically, but there was little evidence of coherence among them; indeed the views of some groups were diametrically opposed to others on fundamental issues, such as the integration of disabled people into society.

These divisions were, and still are, fostered by the State which provides varying types and degrees of provision and benefit on the basis of both impairment and tradition. Oliver and Zarb (1989) believe that this is a deliberate manoeuvre to prevent disabled people from organizing; a strategy on the part of the State to divide and rule.

A large number of disability organizations, controlled by non-disabled people, were also set up at this time; these groups are referred to as organizations *for* disabled people. Some of them date back to the turn of the century or earlier, for example The Royal National Institute for the Blind and the Royal National Institute for the Deaf. Many others were formed in the early years of the Welfare State, for example the Leonard Cheshire Foundation and the Spastics Society. This increase was partly in response to the greater numbers of young disabled people after the Second World War which was due, not only to war injuries, but to the poliomyelitis epidemic of the early 1950s, the Thalidomide episode of the late 1950s and early 1960s, and various medical advances which meant that disabled people survived or lived longer.

With this increase of young disabled people came a proliferation of professionals who, according to Driedger, defined disabled people as 'sick people who spent their lives trying to get well' (1989: 8). It is perhaps ironic that the development of medicine and technology went some way to give disabled people sufficient access to education, employment and community facilities to enable them to organize themselves politically and to challenge the very systems which had made their affiliation possible.

During the 1960s and 1970s organizations of disabled people which crossed impairment boundaries began to develop; the issue which drew them together was poverty. The Disablement Income Group (DIG), formed in 1965 by two disabled women, for example, aimed to secure a disability allowance from the State for all disabled people to compensate them for the extra costs of disability; its appeals and campaigns were notably unsuccessful. This failure, as well as other factors present at the time, including the unfulfilled promises of the 1970 Chronically Sick and Disabled Person's Act, the failure of DIG to tackle the central issues of a disabling environment, the development of the Independent Living Movement in the USA, and the general climate of consumerism and self-help, were all influential in bringing about a shift of focus and a change of mood.

Perhaps the most significant turning point was the formation in 1974 of the Union of the Physically Impaired Against Segregation (UPIAS). Davis (1993) explains how UPIAS fought to change the definition of disability from one of individual tragedy to one of social oppression. It campaigned strongly against the NHS Young Chronic Sick Units which were being built at this time. This emphasis on social oppression paved the way for the development of the social model of disability, which Hasler (1993) refers to as the 'big idea'. The social model of disability encouraged organizations of disabled people to fight collectively for change. Davis believes that 'The birth of UPIAS signalled the end of the welfare-orientated "begging bowl" period and with it the idea that the "experts" could administer away disabled people's problems for them' (1993: 288).

Various innovative projects, underpinned by the social model of disability, commenced during the 1970s. One which was particularly influential was The Grove Road Scheme which was set up in 1979. This scheme was devised by two severely disabled people who wanted to move out of the institution where they lived to get married and set up home together. In the absence of any help from professionals, who thought they were unrealistic, they negotiated a site to build a block of self-contained flats to house disabled and non-disabled people. The flats are run democratically with all residents having an equal say in decision making. The occupants are in contact via an intercom system and, in exchange for payment, the non-disabled residents provide the disabled residents with personal assistance (Davis, 1981).

It is interesting to note that many of the disabled tenants grossly overestimated the amount of assistance they would require from the supporting tenants. The two disabled people who set up the scheme, for example, estimated, on the basis of their experience of institutional care, that together they would need a total of twenty hours assistance per week. In reality they received eight hours of assistance during their first week which dwindled to just an hour and a half per week by the end of the first year. This highlights the way in which institutions create dependency.

Another innovative scheme, started by disabled people at this time, was DIAL UK (Disablement Information and Advice Line) a telephone service aimed to spread straightforward and intelligible information, relating to physical disability, to disabled people and other interested persons. Davis and Woodward contend that 'Information disability is a specific form of social oppression' (1981: 329); the service aimed to eliminate the enormous barriers erected by lack of information in disabled people's lives.

Towards the end of the 1970s the Liberation Network of Disabled People was formed. This had a rather different focus to UPIAS, emphasizing the personal politics of disability and the emancipation of the individual. It will be seen later that this orientation is beginning to re-emerge.

The British Council of Organizations of Disabled People

The United Nations designated 1981 The International Year of Disabled People; it was only after much lobbying that the word *for* was changed to *of*. The working parties involved with this endeavour tended to concentrate on issues defined as important by non-disabled people; there was, for example, a working party on residential care but no such working party on independent living (Hasler, 1993).

In the same year a group of disabled activists, taking advantage of the high profile that the International Year of Disabled People provided, came together to form the British Council of Organization of Disabled People (BCODP) which is an umbrella group for organizations run and controlled by disabled people themselves. UPIAS took the initiative in forming BCODP (Davis and Mullender, 1993). The British Council of Organizations of Disabled People was at first small, representing just 16 organizations, and was initially subjected to a great deal of criticism, with accusations of Marxist leanings and elitism. Pagel states:

> While its formation was welcomed by a large number of disabled people's organisations it was greeted with a degree of hostility by the non-representative, paternalistic charities, who saw it as a challenge to their role as providers for disabled people. (1988: 19)

A large number of BCODP's member organizations comprise coalitions of disabled people and Centres of Integrated Living (see below). Other member organizations include those which focus on specific impairments or single issues, for example The Visually Impaired Teachers and Students Association (VISTA), GEMMA, an organization of disabled lesbians, The Association of Blind Asians, and People First, an organization run by people with learning difficulties. People First and similar organizations of people with learning difficulties, though sharing the goals of other groups within the disability movement, have a different history. They emphasize, in particular, individual and collective empowerment through self-advocacy, self-development, and the expression of feelings and experiences (Simons, 1992).

During the 1980s BCODP grew and continues to expand; it now represents 80 organizations and 200,000 disabled people, and is recognized as the representative voice of disabled people in Great Britain. The major concern of BCODP at the present time is the framing and passing of anti-discrimination legislation; at present there is no such legislation aimed at disabled people in Britain. BCODP articulates its demands through formal political channels and lobbies and advises both central and local government. A recent achievement of BCODP has been the completion and publication of a number of research reports into discrimination (Barnes, 1991), disabling imagery (Barnes, 1992), and independent living (BCODP, 1992). It organizes conferences on topics of interest to disabled people, and in the autumn of 1992 its first journal *Rights not Charity* was launched.

The British Council of Organizations of Disabled People also supports an increasing number of demonstrations and campaigns of direct action; more than a thousand disabled people gathered in October 1992 to express their outrage at the patronizing behaviour and negative imagery portrayed on ITV's Telethon, and the Campaign for Accessible Transport (CAT) frequently engages in protests and acts of civil disobedience. The fact that the courts are generally inaccessible to disabled people who are arrested, serves to reinforce the message of these campaigns. Shakespeare explains the value of direct action:

> Direct action has a number of important elements. It is a way of focusing attention on the institutions and environments that create disability. . . . It is an overtly political act, showing that disability is a matter of social relations, not medical conditions. It is a chance for disabled people to 'do it for themselves' without the help or participation of non-disabled people. . . . It is an empowering process for participants, creating a sense of solidarity, purpose and collective strength which enhances and develops the movement. (1993: 251)

These campaigns and demonstrations appear to have had some success; as Hasler points out 'There was far more media coverage of 12 people sitting down in Oxford Street than 3,000 marching to the DHSS' (1993: 283). The Telethon has, to some extent, improved its imagery of disabled people and its future is now in doubt. The fact that disabled people are able to get together to protest in this way, albeit with difficulty, illustrates some social and environmental improvements, although Hunt reminds us that 'Poverty and inaccessible public transport, institutionalization and years of dependency, were just a few of the limitations disabled people had to work through to establish a collective response' (1992: 60). Rather than being herded together against their will disabled people are now experiencing the exhilaration and liberation of collective action. It would be misleading, however, to portray the disability movement as being free of inner conflict. Some disabled people have expressed concern that, in its struggle for social justice and barrier removal, insufficient attention has been paid to the personal experience of disability (Morris, 1991; Crow, 1992; French, 1993; Handcock, 1993; Keith, 1994). Morris (1991) believes that this tendency to avoid expressing how it feels to be disabled, means that non-disabled people have only their own imaginings to guide them. Shakespeare is concerned about the way in which the disability movement avoids discussion of impairment, he states: 'Given that the majority of unpoliticised disabled people identify first and foremost via their physical impairment, it is an obstacle to their development if this is ignored by the theoreticians of the struggle' (1993: 56). Others believe that BCODP is fashioned and dominated by white men, with the voice of women and black people being barely audible (Hill, 1991; Morris, 1991). Morris states:

> Like other political movements, the disability movement both in Britain and throughout the world, has tended to be dominated by men as both theoreticians and holders of important organisational posts. Both the movement and the development of a theory of disability has been the poorer for this as there has been an accompanying tendency to avoid confronting the personal experience of disability. (1991: 9)

The British Council of Organizations of Disabled People, and the disability movement in general, have been accused of elitism and of failing to represent the views of all disabled people. Oliver (1993) points out, however, that these concerns are rarely raised in relation to other democratic organizations, such as the National Union of Students or the Conservative Party, and objects to the way in which the right of the disability movement to represent disabled people is constantly queried. It is probably the case that the willingness of a disabled elite to associate with other disabled people has been a key factor in the establishment of the disability movement.

Coalitions of disabled people and Centres of Integrated Living

It is mentioned above that a large number of BCODP's member organizations comprise coalitions of disabled people and Centres of Integrated Living (CILs). The first coalition of disabled people in Great Britain was formed in Derbyshire in 1981 and was supported financially by Derbyshire County Council. Various other coalitions, also supported by local government, now exist, including the Manchester Coalition of Disabled People and the Greenwich Coalition of Disabled People.

One of the major activities of these coalitions has been the formation of Centres of Integrated Living (CILs). These centres, which employ many disabled people and base their practice on the social model of disability, gained much of their inspiration and impetus from the Independent Living Movement in the USA which developed in the 1960s and 1970s. The first centre was established in Berkeley California in 1972 and served as a model; at its peak it employed 200 staff and had a budget of $53.2 million. The first centre in Great Britain was the Derbyshire CIL which the Derbyshire Coalition of Disabled People set up in 1985. It expanded rapidly in the late 1980s and at its peak employed 35 people and had a budget of £500,000, though it has since suffered cuts of approximately 50 per cent.

There are important differences between CILs in the USA and those in Great Britain. The main difference is that in Great Britain, owing to the existence of the Welfare State, CILs work in harness with health authorities and local authorities to develop new approaches and to ensure that disabled people receive the support which is their right. Hunt (1992) points out that this arrangement can lead to conflict with the funders. In the USA CILs operate more independently. This difference is reflected in the naming of the centres: in Great Britain they are termed 'Centres of *Integrated* Living', whereas in the USA they are termed 'Centres of *Independent* Living'.

The Derbyshire CIL bases its services around seven basic needs which were identified by the Derbyshire Coalition of Disabled People. These needs are for information, counselling, housing, technical aids, personal assistance, transport and access. Every CIL is unique, but they all provide disabled people with some of these services; a major aim of the centres is to enable severely disabled people to live in the community on their own terms. Other activities of CILs include lobbying members of parliament, advising a wide range of agencies, providing disability equality training, assisting in the framing of legislation, and helping other groups of disabled people to organize politically. The centres offer an explicit critique of prevailing social services based on direct personal experience of disability; many of the early activists had been resident in long-stay institutions themselves. Dougie Herd, convener of the Lothian CIL, states 'The Lothian CIL is, we believe, an example of how the rhetoric of empowerment, user control, and the subtly misnamed "Care in the Community" can be given form and structure which do, indeed, facilitate and encourage disabled people's self-determination' (1992: 21).

Another less obvious function of CILs is to show that disabled people are capable of running their own affairs. As Finkelstein states:

The fact that the centres and the services they provide have been devised and delivered by disabled people also presents a positive and rigorous public image contradicting the general depiction of disabled people as a burden on the state and an appropriate focus for the attention of charity. (1991: 34)

Disabled People's International

Disabled People's International (DPI) was formed in 1981. It represents over 70 national assemblies of disabled people across five continents, including BCODP, and is recognized by the United Nations as the representative body of disabled people internationally (Davis and Mullender, 1993). Disabled People's International grew out of a conflict between disabled and non-disabled people. Until 1981 the only international organization concerned with the needs of people with differing impairments was Rehabilitation International which consisted almost entirely of rehabilitation professionals. A minority of disabled people were, however, involved.

At the 1976 congress of Rehabilitation International, a group of disabled Swedish and Canadian delegates put forward the resolution that at least 50 per cent of the delegation should be representatives of organizations of disabled people. This resolution was strongly defeated which provided the impetus for the 250 disabled people present to form their own organization. Driedger describes the hostility this caused among the rehabilitation professionals, one of whom said:

> To me they are going through a developmental stage which resembles the adolescent or young adult in a family, who often becomes rebellious for a period of time. After this stage, an excellent partnership and relationship with the 'family' evolves and life goes on better than before. (1989: 37)

The relationship between organizations of and organisations for disabled people

From the earliest days of the disability movement, there has been considerable tension and conflict between organizations of and organisations for disabled people. Davis and Mullender state:

> The traditional organisations for disabled people were not about promoting self-organisation, political awareness or control by disabled people over their own lives. Their main role was to alleviate the symptoms rather than relieve the causes of disability. Often they dealt with disabled people's isolation by herding them together in fortnightly

social clubs and taking them on occasional group outings to the seaside. (1993: 7)

Morris (1991) explains that organizations for disabled people have their origins in the surplus time and money of the wealthy. Disability charities also provide many people with a means of earning a living. As Sutherland states 'A considerable number of able-bodied people earn substantial salaries as administrators of charities, while we have the greatest difficulty finding any employment at all. What, then, is that, if not exploitation?' (1981: 117).

Organizations for disabled people are locked into a partnership with the State which operates within an individualistic model of disability and assumes that disabled people cannot take control of their own lives. The influence of the State may also gear charities towards making disabled people economically self-sufficient by training them for or providing them with poorly-paid, low-status employment (Blaxter, 1976). Organizations of disabled people, on the other hand, have their origins in the struggle for civil rights and equality. These tensions and differences of perspective are summed up by Morris who states:

> When the non-disabled society has done things for us it has resulted in our segregation into special schools, residential care and our isolation within a physical, social and economic environment that does not address our needs. Disabled people and their organisations are increasingly insisting that we are the experts on disability and that if we had control over the response to our needs we would develop very different policies from the ones which currently dominate our lives. (1991: 172)

Organizations for disabled people tend to be on the right of the political spectrum and do not, therefore, pose a threat to political, social or economic structures. Organizations of disabled people, on the other hand, tend to be on the left of the political spectrum; their conception of disability as social oppression, especially when it leads to co-operation and collaboration with other marginalized and socially restricted groups, does pose a considerable threat to social order. This may be the reason why organizations of disabled people are so poorly funded when compared with non-representative organizations (Oliver and Zarb, 1989). Oliver (1993) points out that organizations for disabled people receive ten times more funding from central government than organizations of disabled people; in 1990, for example, BCODP received £30,000 from the State whereas The Royal Association of Disability and Rehabilitation (RADAR), the umbrella group of organizations for disabled people, received £500,000. Organizations of disabled people have had to rely on local government for funding, though even this has become severely restricted in recent years.

The dynamic between organizations of and organizations for disabled people is, however, in a state of flux. Although the relationship will never be an easy one, many organizations of and for disabled people do co-operate with each other, and some organizations for disabled people have changed their constitutions to become organizations of disabled people. Even the old traditional charities are beginning to increase the numbers of disabled people on their decision-making bodies.

The disability arts movement

> Choices and rights,
> Choices and rights,
> I want choices and rights in my life.
>
> I don't want your charity,
> Or you to be paid to care for me,
> I want choices and rights in my life.
>
> I don't want to be in your care,
> Or put in some place out there,
> I want choices and rights in my life.
>
> Choices and rights,
> That's what we've got to fight for,
> Choices and rights in my life.
> *Johnnie Creschendo (1990) (singer and songwriter)*

An important element in the struggle of disabled people for equality and social justice is the emergence of the disability arts movement. Disability arts have the power to communicate the distinctive history, skills, customs, experiences and concerns of disabled people, which many believe constitute a distinctive lifestyle and disability culture (Vasey, 1992). The notion of disability culture has been articulated most clearly by the indigenous deaf community (Ladd, 1988), but others, for example Vasey (1992) and Brisenden (1992), have related it to physically disabled people. Brisenden explains 'It is the things we cannot forget as well as the things we want to remember. It is the schools we went to, the day centres we inhabit, but it is also the art we have produced and the organisation we have built. It is so many things but it is no one particular thing' (1992: 63). Brisenden believes that the concept of disability culture has only been made possible by the disability movement.

Disability arts are mainly directed at disabled people themselves.

Most gatherings of disabled people, such as demonstrations, include disabled artists—singers, writers, painters, comedians—who express the experience of disability from their own perspectives, providing alternative, positive, and often overtly heretical ways of viewing disability and society. David Hevey, who describes his contact with the disability movement as 'a flash on the road to Damascus' works as a photographer to 'visualise the politics, celebration and empowerment of disabled people by the disability movement' (1992: 31), and Simon Brisenden (1992), a disabled poet, states that disability arts gave him the one thing he really needed—an audience he could identify with.

It is clear that the disability arts movement can have a profound impact on disabled artists and those who enjoy their work. As Morrison and Finkelstein state 'The arts can have a liberating effect on people . . . having someone on stage communicating ideas and feelings that an isolated disabled person never suspected were shared by others can be a turning point for many' (1993: 27). They go on to explain how the expression of disability culture in art can give disabled people a voice and a valid role to play in the disability movement. It also helps to negate any tendency for the disability movement to be controlled by an elite.

There are now several theatre companies of disabled people, the most famous being Graeae, and various disability arts publications, including Disability Arts in London (DAIL) and Disability Arts Magazine (DAM). As well as presenting the work of disabled artists, these magazines give details of events such as signed theatre, disabled cabaret, and exhibitions of the work of disabled artists.

The notion of disability culture can be deeply threatening to non-disabled people, as well as disabled people who have achieved assimilation in the 'normal' world. This is because it challenges the cultural representations of disability and gives disabled people as much worth and value as other members of society. As Oliver states, 'cultural expressions of the disability movement provide a challenge to the stigmatization of difference in its insistence that disability is a cause for celebration' (1993: 26). Celebrating disability may also give rise to feelings of insecurity in non-disabled people.

Conclusion

> From the celebration of our difference and shared experience, great movements and a better world can evolve. (Woolley, 1993: 83)

Hasler (1993) believes that the disability movement has changed the discourse on disability by redefining its meaning, and Wood (1990) is of the opinion that the disability movement has had 'a massive effect' on local authorities, health authorities and the professions, as well as exerting considerable influence on central government. Hunt (1992) is more cautious, however, pointing out that although public attitudes have changed the disability movement still lacks power.

Perhaps the most important achievement of the disability movement is the powerful impact it has had on disabled people themselves. Disabled people have been internally oppressed by their conditioning. This has given rise to negative feelings about themselves and other disabled people, similar to those held by the non-disabled world (Mason, 1992b). One of the major achievements of the disability movement is the support it offers disabled people in ridding themselves of this oppression.

History is harsh in teaching that all oppressed groups must engage in struggle for their rights (Coleridge, 1993). Munro and Elder-Woodward (1992) point out that people can only fight for their rights when they are aware of their oppression; the active engagement in struggle is a crucial part of this consciousness raising process. As Oliver states:

> It is often assumed that empowerment is a process by which those in society who have power can dispense some of their power to those who don't have any. . . . However, it is more realistic to see empowerment as a collective process on which the powerless embark as part of their struggle to resist the oppression of others and/or to articulate their own views of the world. (Oliver 1993: 24)

Disability is now recognized by disabled people as a civil rights issue, and the stigma attached to disability, which has served as such a powerful disincentive to 'coming out', is gradually being eroded.

Pagel (1988) believes that professionals working with disabled people are being presented with a choice; on the one hand they can continue to contribute to the oppression faced by disabled people or, on the other, they can alter their practices and services to help and support disabled people as they strive to achieve equal status with other members of society. Disabled people are already working in partnership with professionals who have chosen the second course.

References

Abercrombie, N., Hill, S. and Turner, B. (1988) *Dictionary of Sociology*, Penguin Books, Harmondsworth

Barnes, C. (1991) *Disabled People in Britain and Discrimination*, Hurst & Company, London

Barnes, C. (1992) *Disabling Imagery and the Media*, The British Council of Organizations of Disabled People and Ryburn Publishing Limited, Halifax

Blaxter, M. (1976) *The Meaning of Disability*, Heinemann, London

Brisenden, S. (1992) What is disability culture? In *Disability Equality in the Classroom: A Human Rights Issue*, (eds B. Rieser and M. Mason), Disability Equality in Education, London

British Council of Organizations of Disabled People (1992) Independence '92: a report from BCODP on the workshops held in Vancouver, Canada, 22–26 April, 1992

Coleridge, P. (1993) *Disability, Liberation, and Empowerment*, Oxfam, Oxford

Creschendo, J. (1990) Video of the disability equality pack: *Disability— Changing Practice* (K665x), Open University, Milton Keyes

Crow, L. (1992) Renewing the social model of disability, *Coalition*, July, Greater Manchester Coalition of Disabled People, 5–9

Davis, K. (1981) 28–38 Grove Road: accommodation and care in a community setting. In *Handicap in a Social World*, (eds A. Brechin, P. Liddiard and J. Swain), Hodder & Stoughton. Sevenoaks

Davis, K. (1993) On the Movement. In *Disabling Barriers—Enabling Environments*, (eds J. Swain, V. Finkelstein, S. French and M. Oliver), Sage, London

Davis, K. and Mullender, A. (1993) *Ten Turbulent Years: A review of the Work of the Derbyshire Coalition of Disabled People*, The Derbyshire Coalition of Disabled People and The Centre for Social Action, University of Nottingham

Davis, K. and Woodward, J. (1981) DIAL UK: development of the National Association of Disablement Information and Advice Services. In *Handicap in a Social World*, (eds A. Brechin, P. Liddiard and J. Swain), Hodder & Stoughton, Sevenoaks

Driedger, D. (1989) *The Last Civil Rights Movement*, Hurst & Company, London

Enticott, J., Graham, P. and Lamb, B. (1992) *Polls Apart: Disabled People and the 1992 General Election*, The Spastics Society, London

Finkelstein, V. (1991) Disability: an administrative challenge. In *Social Work, Disabled People and Disabling Environments*, (ed. M. Oliver), Jessica Kingsley, London

French, S. (1993) Disability, impairment or something in between? In *Disabling Barriers—Enabling Environments*, (eds J. Swain, V. Finkelstein, S. French and M. Oliver), Sage, London

Giddens, A. (1989) *Sociology*, Polity Press, Cambridge

Handcock, S. (1993) Disability and loss—is it a taboo subject? *Boadicea*, February/March, **3**, 1

Hasler, F. (1993) Developments in the disabled people's movement. In *Disabling Barriers—Enabling Environments*, (eds J. Swain, V. Finkelstein, S. French and M. Oliver), Sage, London

Herd, D. (1992) Cited in Centres for Independent Living, *Rights not Charity*, **1 (2)**, 19–21

Hevey, D. (1992) *The Creatures Time Forgot: Photography and Disability Imagery*, Routledge, London

Hill, M. (1991) Race and disability. In the book of readings of the disability equality pack *Disability—Identity, Sexuality and Relationships* (K665y), Open University, Milton Keynes

Hunt, J. (1992) The disabled people's movement between 1960–1986 and its effect upon the development of community support services. M Sc Dissertation by independent study, University of East London

Keith, L. (ed.) (1994) *Mustn't Grumble: writing by disabled women*, The Women's Press, London

Ladd, P. (1988) The modern deaf community. In *British Sign Language*, (ed. D. Miles), BBC Books, London

Mason, M. (1992a) The disability movement. In *Disability Equality in the Classroom: A Human Rights Issue*, (2nd edn) (eds R. Rieser and M. Mason), Disability Equality in Education, London

Mason, M. (1992b) Internalised Oppression. In *Disability Equality in the Classroom: A Human Rights Issue*, (2nd edn) (eds R. Rieser and M. Mason), Disability Equality in Education, London

Morris, J. (1991) *Pride Against Prejudice*, The Women's Press, London

Morris, J. (1992) Feminism and disability, *Feminist Review*, Spring, **43**, 57–70

Morrison, E. and Finkelstein, V. (1993) Broken arts and cultural repair: the role of culture in the empowerment of disabled people. In *Disabling Barriers—Enabling Environments* (eds J. Swain, V. Finkelstein, S. French and M. Oliver), Sage, London

Munro, K. and Elder-Woodward, J. (1992) *Independent Living*, Churchill Livingstone, Edinburgh

Oliver, M. (1990) *The Politics of Disablement*, Macmillan, London

Oliver, M. (1993) Disability, citizenship and empowerment. Workbook 2 of the course *The Disabling Society* (K665), Open University, Milton Keynes

Oliver, M. and Zarb, G. (1989) The politics of disability: a new approach. *Disability, Handicap and Society*, **4 (5)**, 221–239

Pagel, M. (1988) *On Our Own Behalf*, Greater Manchester Coalition of Disabled People, Manchester

Shakespeare, T. (1993) Disabled people's self-organisation: a new social movement? *Disability, Handicap and Society*, **8 (3)**, 249–264

Simons, K. (1992) *'Sticking Up for Yourself' Self-advocacy and People with Learning Difficulties*, Joseph Rowntree Foundation, London

Sutherland, A. T. (1981) *Disabled We Stand*, Souvenir Press, London

Vasey, S. (1992) Disability culture: it's a way of life. In *Disability Equality in the Classroom: A Human Rights Issue*, (eds R. Rieser and M. Mason), Disability Equality in Education, London

Wood, R. (1990) The British Council of Organizations of Disabled People—our history. In *Building Our lives*, (ed. L. Laurie), Shelter, London

Woolley, M. (1993) Acquired hearing loss: acquired oppression. In *Disabling Barriers—Enabling Environments*, (eds J. Swain, V. Finkelstein, S. French and M. Oliver), Sage, London

PART TWO

WORKING WITH DISABLED PEOPLE

7

Learning about disability: changing attitudes or challenging understanding?

John Swain and Paul Lawrence

Introduction

Our general focus in this chapter is on training in 'disability' for nurses and therapists. In particular, we shall be exploring the issues that arise for both those who provide and receive training and staff development programmes, issues which come under the umbrella of 'evaluation'. As McCormack and Kenefick point out in their book about 'new approaches to training and development in disability services': 'There is a great and growing array of courses, seminars and workshops available from the universities, specialist agencies and individual training consultants' (1991: 15). We shall concentrate here on 'disability awareness/equality training', that is programmes of study which are specifically aimed at changing attitudes and behaviour towards disabled people.

Courses are evaluated in many ways, both formally and informally. This can include, for instance, an evaluation form which is completed by course participants with questions which can range from 'did you enjoy it?' to 'was it useful in your work?'. Course providers are under increasing pressure to be accountable to their 'clients' at every stage of planning and evaluating courses. The questions which can be raised are far reaching.

1. What is it that health professionals should be made aware of? What are the overall aims of the course?
2. What is meant by 'disability' on the course? What understanding is conveyed in the materials and processes of teaching and learning?
3. What do we mean by 'awareness'? Does this cover understanding, attitudes, behaviour or maybe even skills?

4. What constitutes and is effective 'training'? How should profes-
    sionals learn about disability?
5. What is the content or syllabus of disability training?
6. Who are the learners and who are the trainers?

It is these questions which provide the starting point for our discussions. By exploring these issues we hope to facilitate nurses, therapists, their tutors and course providers in critically examining the
process of 'learning about disability'.

An attitude problem

The notion of 'disability awareness training' has a lengthy history. It
has its roots in beliefs that the integration and participation of disabled people in communities is limited by the negative attitudes they
face. The need for programmes of disability awareness training, including for members of the public and professionals, is closely associated with moves from institutional to community care (McConkey
and McCormack, 1983). Florian and Kehat put the argument succinctly in a more recent statement:

> the negative social attitudes that exist in almost every community
> toward people with disabilities remain a major obstacle to the social
> reintegration and rehabilitation of those who are disabled. (1987: 57)

'Attitudes' are, however, complex. They are generally seen as having
three aspects: first, a cognitive component, that is knowledge and
understanding of 'disability' (this can include knowledge of terms
such as impairment, disability and handicap; knowledge of medical
conditions and so on); second, an emotional component, that is the
feelings provoked by disabled people; and third, a behavioural component, that is how people act and react towards disabled people.
Attitudes are complicated further because there is a loose connection
between these three components. Our understanding, our feelings
and what we do about things do not necessarily relate closely to each
other. For example we can feel very strongly about something but not
do anything about it. Nevertheless, each of the components is seen to
play a part in negative attitudes. A negative attitude to people with
Down's Syndrome might include, for instance, a lack of understanding about the medical condition (eg it is seen as a form of mental
illness), a fear of people with Down's Syndrome (eg not knowing how
to respond) and a behaviour component such as name calling and
negative labelling (eg 'mongol'). Professionals, including those in the
health field, are seen as possible contributors to such attitudes.

Of the three components of attitudes the most commonly cited seem to be emotional aspects. Roush's statement is a recent example:

> Typical emotional reactions when seeing someone with a disability include guilt, fear, and pity, all of which are characterised by a general feeling of discomfort. (1986: 1551)

Such prejudice has been written about by some disabled people themselves, including Morris:

> Although overt hostility is not a common experience for most disabled people, it is yet the iron fist in the velvet glove of the patronising and seemingly benevolent attitudes which we experience. This is clear from the experiences of those of us who step out of the passive role which our society accords to us. In these situations we often have to confront dislike, revulsion and fear. (1993: 103)

This, then, has been the basis for many programmes and studies. They differ in terms of their stated aims (which of the three components is given priority); their audience; their methods; and their criteria for evaluating effectiveness. There are three basic approaches, though a combination is often used.

1. Information and education programmes
   These involve the provision of 'information' through the use of such things as fact sheets, discussions, photographs, videos and lecture sessions. For instance, in the provision of disability awareness training to facilitate the integration of disabled students in colleges of further education, Chapman recommends the provision of information about specific disabilities, about adaptations and aids that might be of value to staff or students, and advice about ways in which teaching strategies may be adapted to meet the needs of a disabled student (1986: 12).
2. Role play and simulation exercises
   These involve such activities as role playing situations involving disabled people and simulating various impairments such as blindness through the use of blindfolds.
3. Contact with disabled people
   This again can take a variety of forms including: 'unobserved or unobtrusive staring'; the use of disabled people as visiting lecturers; visits to institutions (such as special schools); sharing informal social activities.

The three approaches can be related to the three components of attitudes (Florian and Kehat, 1987). Thus information can be seen as influencing the cognitive component, role play and simulation the emotional side, and contact primarily behaviour. Whatever the differences, however, all such programmes and studies share the general

aim of changing the attitudes of non-disabled people, and a significant amount of energy, resources and effort has been invested.

In the face of this investment the whole notion of 'disability awareness training' based on changing attitudes has been challenged in
many ways, particularly by disabled people and their organizations.
Perhaps the first note of warning came from research studies themselves which showed that even in their own terms programmes did
not necessarily work. In terms of attitudes generally, it has been
believed for many years that 'attitudes are relatively stable' (McDavid
and Harari, 1968: 131). In relation to disability, as far back as the late
1960s Wilson and Alcorn (1969) found that a programme to change
attitudes was ineffective. They subjected groups of college students
to exercises which simulated blindness, deafness and mobility impairment, through the use of wheelchairs, blindfolds and so on. They
found no significant difference, on a measure of 'Attitudes Towards
Disabled Persons', between the experimental group and a control
group who had not undertaken the programme.

Such findings have been taken into account by some advocates of
attitude changing programmes. Both Wright (1980) and McConkey
and McCormack (1983) argue that some particular techniques used in
certain ways are more effective than others. They suggest that contact
with disabled people is more likely to change the attitudes of non–
disabled people, for instance, when both groups meet as equals (eg
they are of similar ages and have similar interests) and there is
personal contact. Wright argues for 'coping versus succumbing
frameworks' (1980: 275). From her stand-point it is not the general
direction which is wrong but the techniques which are used. The
whole programme should be geared towards seeing disabled people
as active participants in their own lives and in the life of the community. Thus disability simulation should enable non-disabled people to
discover that, for instance, it is possible to live with blindness because
the blind person actively seeks to deal with the problems of living and
learns techniques of management. The focus is on the person as a
person, rather than disability, the environmental changes necessary
for disabled people to live a better quality of life, and the possible
change for the disabled person through medical and psychological
procedures. She argues that:

> Constructive views of life with a disability, conceptualized within the
> coping framework, provide an excellent basis for developing positive
> attitudes.
>
> One example of a constructive view is that people with disabilities are
> not passive—they do and must actively take charge of their lives, they
> are highly differentiated as individuals. (1980: 279)

For Wright then it is the nature of the picture that is painted which matters. To change attitudes in a positive direction it must be a positive picture.

French (1992) has developed another line of critique, in relation to simulation exercises, which goes beyond the idea that programmes may not work to suggest that they can actually be counter-productive. Her main points are as follows.

1. Simulation exercises provide false information about the situation of disabled people. For instance, impairment is only a temporary state for non-disabled people. They remove the blindfold and they are sighted again. Furthermore, disabled people develop all kinds of strategies which cannot be 'simulated' in such exercises.
2. Simulation exercises, by their very nature, focus on supposed difficulties, problems, inadequacies and inabilities of disabled people. They contribute to rather than challenge damaging stereotypes.
3. What is being simulated is impairment not disability. The whole orientation is on people's feelings about impairment rather than the barriers and oppression faced by disabled people.

The most fundamental of all the challenges towards disability awareness training questions the theoretical stance which is being taken. Most of the literature which documents an 'attitudes changing' approach has little to say about the possible sources of supposed negative attitudes. However, three general theories seem to be prevalent (Livneh, 1982). The first holds that negative attitudes are grounded in an innate or instinctual fear, that is a fear of impairment along the same lines as a fear of death. The second assumes that negative attitudes arise from perceived psychological threat, conscious or unconscious such as the fear of supposed loss of value of property if disabled people move into a neighbourhood. The third theory points to societal norms, beliefs and values which discourage non-disabled people from associating or having contact with disabled people. All these theories explain attitudes in terms of reactions to disabled people, and in particular difference and impairment. As Abberley argues, there is no 'attempt to specify why particular ideas are held in particular societies at particular times' (1993: 110). Attitudes are seen as separate from their whole historical and social context, and as ultimately caused by disabled people. If only they were not 'abnormal' there would be no negative attitudes. Furthermore, again as Abberley points out, such theoretical positions promote a pessimistic prognosis for disabled people. Negative attitudes are founded upon reactions to impairment and thus all the energy and effort to change them can only be cosmetic.

It is in this light that organizations of disabled people have rejected the whole notion of 'disability awareness training', aimed at changing attitudes, as being misconceived and misdirected. What is required, essentially, is a questioning of the meaning of 'disability' which is directed and conceived by disabled people themselves. It is this challenging of understanding to which we shall now turn.

Redefining 'the problem'

The whole notion of 'disability equality training' has quite different roots from that of 'disability awareness training'. As we shall discuss later, this distinction is not quite so clear-cut as it sounds, but in general terms there are some clear distinctions between the two. Disability equality training:

- is about disability rather than about impairment;
- is about challenging understanding of 'disability', and changing practices, rather than about improving general attitudes towards disabled people;
- promotes a social rather than an individual tragedy model of disability;
- is seen as part of the wider struggle for equal opportunities in both policies and practices (for women, black and minority ethnic people and lesbians and gays);
- uses discussion-based methods for teaching and learning rather than simulation;
- is devised and delivered by disabled people.

In its strictest sense disability equality training refers to courses delivered only by tutors who have been trained by organizations of disabled people, in particular the London Boroughs Disability Resource Team (now called simply the Disability Resource Team) and the Greater Manchester Coalition of Disabled People. These organizations train disabled people themselves to be trainers. The courses are not about changing attitudes towards disabled people but about challenging people's whole understanding of the meaning of 'disability'. The following are the stated aims of courses run by disabled trainers who have themselves been trained through the work of the London Boroughs Disability Resources Team:

> A D.E.T. course will enable participants to identify and address discriminatory forms of practice towards disabled people. Through training they will find ways to challenge the organisational behaviour which reinforces negative myths and values and which prevents disabled people from gaining equality and achieving full participation in society. (Gillespie-Sells and Campbell, 1991: 9)

These are mainly short, two-day courses, which are devised and run for specific groups of people, particularly distinct groups of professionals, including nurses and therapists. They do not involve simulation or 'contact with disabled people' where such contact is devised as a part of the course. They are rather, however, planned and run by disabled people. As Gillespie-Sells and Campbell state, 'only those who experience disability as a form of social oppression really understand thoroughly enough to teach about its reality' (1991: 7). The training methods used are primarily based on discussions around case studies, role play, videos and other materials. These techniques are used to explore disability as an equal opportunities issue, *not* impairment. The content of the courses covers such topics as redefining disability, images of disability, understanding links and parallels with other oppressed groups and community care and the social model of disability.

The roots of disability equality training lie in the politicizing of disability issues. The focus is not on 'disability' as a condition of the individual but on the barriers faced in a society geared by and for non-disabled people: barriers which exclude disabled people from full active citizenship. These barriers can permeate every aspect of the physical and social environment: attitudes, institutions, language and culture, organization and delivery of support services, and the power relations and structures which constitute society. Disability equality training is about the different forms of institutional discrimination which disabled people face. It is essentially about redefining 'disability'. Arguments over definitions are often reduced to supposedly technical purposes, but they are in effect part of the struggle to establish and legitimate one way of thinking over another. Definitions of disability are themselves part of the creation and maintenance of barriers or enabling environments. The establishment of definition is central to clarifying the route to full citizenship.

There are two crucial points in terms of the effectiveness of disability equality training. The first is the control by disabled people. Disability, and how it is overcome, is defined by disabled people: their understandings, their intentions, and their desires. The transformation of power relations is fundamental to overcoming disabling barriers and establishing enabling environments (Swain et al., 1993). This involves the establishment of equal opportunities and support for the emancipation of disabled people.

The second point is that, in establishing support, disability equality training needs to permeate to a wide audience. Barnes, for instance, gives examples of architectural barriers which could easily be overcome through increased disability awareness training among architects and planners. Similarly he suggests that:

there should be heightened involvement of all personnel throughout the media, including broadcasting companies, newspapers and advertising agencies, in comprehensive disability awareness training courses designed and presented by disabled people. (1991: 204).

French (1993a) argues that there is a need for the general public and, in particular the staff who work on public transport systems, to receive disability equality training. Perhaps the priority, given their position in the power structures which dominate the lives of disabled people, is disability equality training for professionals. Butterworth (1988) argues, for instance, that community nurses should become politically aware and politically involved in disability issues. Such awareness and involvement is a goal of disability equality training.

Finally in this section it should be said that disabled people have been engaged in numerous activities around the country which, while they could not be called disability equality training in the strict sense we have pursued so far, do have many of the essential features (not least being controlled by disabled people). Sutcliffe (1990) has documented a number of examples particularly involving people with learning difficulties. These include the Strathcona Theatre Company who write and perform their own plays. Amongst other things, they have worked with fourth year medical students challenging them to examine their own attitudes and responses to disability. Many other activities by disabled people could be included here as contributing to disability equality training, such as: the development of Disability Arts (for instance, 'The Ghetto', an international disability cabaret which appeared at the 1993 Edinburgh Arts Festival); and the campaigns and demonstrations of the Disability Movement (for instance against 'Telethon'). (For further information on the disability movement and the disability arts movement, the reader is referred to chapter 6.)

'Understanding Disability' and 'Disability—Changing Practice': two examples of disability awareness/equality training programmes

The issues in evaluating 'learning about disability' are, then, highly complex. The aims and actual messages which come across in training and staff development for nurses and therapists can even be contradictory. To further the process of critical questioning, we shall look at two specific examples of disability training programmes. The first is *Understanding Disability* (UD), published in 1993 by Understanding Disability Educational Trust (Weydon School, Weydon Lane,

Farnham, Surrey GU9 8UG); and the second *Disability—Changing Practice* (CP) published in 1990 by the Open University (Central Enquiry Service, PO Box 71, Walton Hall, Milton Keynes MK7 6AG). We have selected these two for discussion as they are both readily available and because they are recent developments. They also contain the types of materials and exercises which health professionals may well encounter in their training and staff development.

The UD programme is covered in 12 to 13 sessions presented in 4 units of study:

Disability and Physical Impairment;
Disability and Hearing Impairment;
Disability and Learning Impairment;
Disability and Visual Impairment.

For each unit there are teaching notes, a video and a set of supporting resources. Disabled people participated in the production of the programme and the materials, which seem to be firmly grounded in the experiences and views of disabled people. Furthermore, the experiences of disabled people are directly reflected in the course, by disabled people talking on video or being invited as 'guests' to discuss issues with the course members. The pack was originally designed for students of 16+ but we have used some of the materials on an in-service course for health care workers.

The CP package is intended to be flexible and can be studied either by an individual or within a group. It consists of 8 sessions which can be presented in a two-day workshop. The materials include a home study text, a booklet of readings, group leader's notes, two audio cassettes and a video. The course was devised for the Open University by a course team led by Vic Finkelstein who has been a political activist and a leading figure in the disability movement for many years. The course is 'concerned with raising awareness about the key issues involved in removing the barriers to the full integration of disabled people into their communities' (Finkelstein, 1990: 9). It was designed for anyone working with disabled people (statutory services or voluntary organizations), disabled people themselves and close relatives.

There is much that is ostensibly similar between these two programmes. Both can be more easily identified with disability equality training than disability awareness training, in the terms that they were distinguished above (though both use the word 'awareness'). Both are concerned with challenging understanding, both eschew the use of simulation activities (though the Understanding Disability Educational Trust made extensive use of such activities in their previously published programmes), and both wish to promote a social model of disability. It is the central role of the social model which we shall look at in more detail in order to review the general message being portrayed and the implications for change.

The stated aim for the UD programme is as follows:

> This course has been designed to develop an understanding that society's prevailing attitudes and the environment often cause unnecessary disability to people with impairments. An informed awareness can lead to environmental changes allowing disabled people greater independence, opportunity and choice. Each aspect of the course, especially the active participation of disabled guests, encourages patronising notions to be dispelled e.g. mistaken ideas ('No blind person can see anything at all'), hurtful vocabulary ('spazzo') and unthinking behaviour ('Does he take sugar?') (Understanding Disability Educational Trust, 1993: 2)

The programme, then, aims to develop awareness of the social and physical barriers experienced by disabled people and 'disability awareness' is defined in terms of understanding a social model of disability. A 'social model' of disability is espoused in which disability is defined in terms of and located within society rather than the individual. The course designers cite the most widely quoted source for a social model of disability, that is the classifications proposed by the Union of the Physically Impaired Against Segregation (UPIAS):

> *Impairment* lacking part of or all of a limb, or having a defective limb, organism or mechanism of the body;
> *Disability* the disadvantage or restriction of activity caused by a contemporary social organisation which takes no or little account of people who have physical impairments and thus excludes them from the mainstream of social activities. (UPIAS, 1976: 3–4)

The CP course is likewise concerned with raising questions about how disability is perceived, including the following:

1. how we use disability-related words such as 'impairment' and 'handicap' and what we mean by these words in different contexts;
2. how barriers (environmental, structural and attitudinal) which restrict the opportunity for people to participate in the activities of daily living, not only affect their lives but also disable them;
3. how positive action needs to be implemented to ensure equal opportunities for disabled people in education, employment, leisure and as members of society. (Finkelstein, 1990: 11)

Despite the similarities, there are significant differences between the two in terms of the social model presented. First, the model as presented in the UD programme is not to any great extent viewed as part of the struggle of the disability movement to establish and legitimate one way of thinking over another. As Oliver states:

> A social theory of disability, however, must be located within the experience of disabled people themselves and their attempts, not only to redefine disability but also to construct a political movement amongst themselves and to develop services commensurate with their own self-defined needs. (1990: 11)

Seen in this way, the social model of disability is integral to the social movement of disabled people. Yet in this programme the political nature of the social model is given little attention. For instance, during the whole of the video and accompanying notes dealing with physical impairment no mention is made of the growth of groups of disabled people or of the disability movement, except in the form of one short note. All the barriers are shown as being faced by individuals and sometimes overcome by individuals.

On the other hand, the CP programme, even in the 'welcome to the course', discusses redefinitions and changing understanding in the context of the rapid growth of organizations of disabled people and their struggle to remove the barriers to integration. Furthermore, many examples are provided of the role of self-help groups of disabled people, such as in the development of Centres for Integrated Living to provide community-based services for disabled people.

Second, the relationship between categorization of people by impairment, as in the structure of the UD programme, and the social model of disability is problematic. As Oliver states:

> An adequate social theory of disability as social restriction must reject categories based upon medical or social scientific constructions and divorced from the direct experience of disabled people. (Oliver, 1990: xiii–xiv)

The divisive consequences of such systems of categorization can be seen in the video programmes. For instance Steven, a young disabled person, affirms his identity by denial of supposed learning difficulties: 'it doesn't mean that I haven't got the brain power' and 'the idea that we're stupid hasn't gone.' The implication being, of course, that all the negative attitudes and social barriers he faces would be justified if he *was* a person with learning difficulties.

This is an issue which receives some discussion within the CP package. Though it is recognized that there is some rivalry between disability groups it is suggested that 'the themes discussed are considered to be equally relevant to all disability groups.' Students are, however, left to 'exercise their minds' when relating the themes to the experiences of different disability groups.

The third set of questions invoke some highly complex issues which we can only touch on here. The key to the social model is reflected in the aims of both these programmes. Crow encapsulates its importance for disabled people:

> The social model was the explanation I had sought for years. Suddenly what I had always known, deep down, was confirmed. It wasn't my body that was responsible for all my difficulties, it was external factors. I was being Dis-abled—my capabilities and opportunities were being restricted—by poor social organisation. Even more important, if all the problems have been created by society, then surely society could un-create them. Revolutionary! (1992: 5)

And it is this revolution which disability equality training pursues. Yet there are variations, some subtle and some quite fundamental, between what are described as 'social models'. Morris, for instance, argues from the viewpoint of a disabled feminist writer (see also French, 1993b). Writing of the domination of the disability movement by men she states:

> Both the movement and the development of a theory of disability has been the poorer for this as there has been an accompanying tendency to avoid confronting the personal experience of disability. (Morris, 1991: 70)

From this perspective, the social model of disability adhered to in the programme means that the experiences of many people who see themselves as disabled are neglected or denied. Experiences of pain, for instance, are difficult to equate with environmental barriers and are not discussed during the programme. Crow argues that:

> What we need to do is take a fresh look at the social model and learn to integrate all its complexities. . . . We need to focus on disability and impairment: on the external and internal constituents they bring to our experiences. (1992: 8)

So what part does impairment play in the social models of disability as reflected in the two programmes we are considering here? In UD it is not clear. Though a social understanding of disability is empha-sized, the pack does provide summaries of some medical conditions 'causing physical impairment' in appendices as information for the tutor in case of questions 'about specific conditions'. Here there are inconsistencies in their particular 'social model'. For instance, cerebral palsy is referred to as a 'physical disability' which 'can be accompa-nied by a learning disability'. Thus, despite the stated intentions of the pack, this reflects a medical rather than a social model of disability.

CP provides no such list of medical conditions. An interactive approach is taken in which disability is regarded as 'the outcome of an interaction between particular types of body impairment and the way the social and physical environment is constructed' (Finkelstein, 1990: 22). Thus even in programmes which use a social model of disability there can be important differences between the precise details of the models pursued.

Both the programmes are geared towards challenging people's understanding of disability, but how is this related to social change for disabled people? The UD pack states:

> By placing an emphasis on the social, rather than the medical aspects of disability, changes in attitude and the environment will increase opportunity, independence and choice for disabled people. (Understanding Disability Awareness Trust, 1993: 3)

Particular examples are provided in the introduction to the teaching pack as follows:

> e.g. access to a physically disabled person may be denied because of the built environment, but access to a learning or sensory impaired person may be denied as a result of their communication needs not being met. Both these situations could be overcome if there was greater disability awareness in society. (Understanding Disability Educational Trust, 1993: 3)

What is being changed, then, is attitudes. In particular it is the cognitive dimension of attitudes which is concentrated on, in the hope that changes in behaviour will follow changes in understanding. In this respect, the most general criticism which can be levelled against such disability awareness/equality training is that it is long on understanding and short on prescription or what to do about it. Furthermore, the processes of social change do not seem to have been considered in the design of this programme. How is change to be brought about in the built environment, for instance, and who instigates such a change?

In the CP course the pressures for change are more clearly identified: change comes from disabled people themselves defining and working towards the removal of barriers that they face in the community. In the group sessions participants are asked in one activity to consider how the course

> might lead to changes in individual practice in ways of working, ways of talking about and to disabled people, and ways of devising and following administrative procedures (assessment, writing up notes, making referrals). (Dant and Quinn 1990: 42)

It has to be said, however, that the implications for changing practice are not further developed.

Conclusion: questions of evaluation

We shall conclude by drawing together what we see as the three main sets of issues with regard to evaluating courses/programmes for learning about disability. These are concerns for all involved, including nurses and therapists as course participants as well as tutors and designers of courses.

The first focus for evaluation, one we have pursued in this chapter, is the course itself. This begins with the stated aims and whether the course adheres to a 'personal tragedy' model which concentrates on the individual disabled person (medical conditions, impairments, their problems and abilities or inabilities, and so on) or a 'social model' which concentrates on the social and physical environment (the barriers to participation, unequal rights, discrimination and so on). The next set of questions concerns the reflection of this orientation in every aspect of the teaching and learning process, the materials, processes of evaluation within the course, and reading list. Such questions need to be posed even if there are no stated aims for the course.

Still more difficult issues arise with regard to the contributions of 'learning about disability' to processes of social change. In terms of changing the practice of professionals in particular, questions can be asked about the relationship between a short programme of disability awareness training, of this nature, and the whole of the training courses provided for health professionals. The *Understanding Disability* pack, for instance, eschews the medical model, stating that the 'group should not be overwhelmed by biological and medical facts' (though medical conditions are described in appendices, as mentioned above). Yet it is such 'facts' which are the mainstay of the health professionals' training. Such 'facts' are the major component of the course content, the basis for assessment and professional certification and, ultimately, part of the justification of the professional's role and status. The question of the role of disability awareness/equality training, based on a social model of disability, within the whole training programme for health professionals remains problematic. Furthermore, as Finkelstein points out:

> Therapists who teach about disability yet have no direct experience of working with a disabled person as a colleague will lack important information about what it is possible for disabled people to accomplish. They will be inclined to hold on to the view that disabled people, as a social group, are basically people in need of care and support. (1990: 30)

Finally, while there has been, as we discussed above, a good deal of research into attitudes towards disabled people, particularly negative emotional reactions to impairments, there has been little research into attitudes towards the disabling physical and social environment. As Oliver states:

> The urgent task for research, and indeed researchers, is to create an epistemology and methodology which takes as its starting-point the central idea that disability is socially created. (1993: 65)

He goes on to say that:

> The crucial point to be made is that these developments can only be facilitated by establishing a partnership between researchers and disabled people, for neither can do it alone. (1993: 65)

References

Abberley, P. (1993), Disabled people and 'normality'. In *Disabling Barriers—Enabling Environments*, (eds J. Swain, V. Finkelstein, S. French and M. Oliver), Sage, London

Barnes, C. (1991) *Disabled People in Britain and Discrimination: A Case for Anti-discrimination Legislation*, Hurst & Company, London

Butterworth, T. (1988) Political awareness. *Community*, December, 20–21

Chapman, L. (1986) The provision of in-house disability awareness training for staff in colleges. *Educare*, **26**, 12–17

Crow, L. (1992) Renewing the Social Model of Disability. *Coalition*, Greater Manchester Coalition of Disabled People, July, 5–9

Dant, T. and Quinn, G. (1990) *Group leader notes*, K665X, *Disability—Changing Practice*, Open University Press, Milton Keynes

Finkelstein, V. (1990) *Home study text*, K665X, *Disability—Changing Practice*, Open University Press, Milton Keynes

Florian, V. and Kehat, D. (1987) Changing high school students' attitudes towards disabled people. *Health and Social Work*, **12 (1)** 57–63

French, S. (1992) Simulation exercises in disability awareness training. *Disability, Handicap and Society*, **7 (3)**, 257–266

French, S. (1993a) *Dismantling the barriers*, Workbook 3 K665, *The Disabling Society*, Open University Press, Milton Keynes

French, S. (1993b) Disability, impairment or something in between? In *Disabling Barriers—Enabling Environments*, (eds J. Swain, V. Finkelstein, S. French and M. Oliver), Sage, London

Gillespie-Sills, K. and Campbell, J. (1991) *Disability Equality Training: Trainers Guide*, Central Council for Education and Training in Social Work, London

Livneh, H. (1982) On the origin of negative attitudes towards people with disabilities. *Rehabilitation Literature*, **43**, 11–12

McConkey, R. and McCormack, B. (1983) *Breaking Barriers: Educating People about Disability*, Souvenir Press, London

McCormack, B. and Kenefick, D. (1991) *Learning On The Job: New Approaches to Training and Development in Disability Services*, Souvenir Press, London

McDavid, J. W. and Harari, H. (1968) *Social Psychology*, Harper International, London

Morris, J. (1991) *Pride Against Prejudice: Transforming Attitudes to Disability*, The Women's Press, London

Morris, J. (1993) Prejudice. In *Disabling Barriers—Enabling Environments*, (eds J. Swain, V. Finkelstein, S. French and M. Oliver), Sage, London

Oliver, M. (1990) *The Politics of Disablement*, Macmillan, Basingstoke

Oliver, M. (1993) Re-defining disability: a challenge to research. In *Disabling Barriers—Enabling Environments*, (eds J. Swain, V. Finkelstein, S. French and M. Oliver), Sage, London

Open University (1990) K665x, *Disability—Changing Practice*, Open University Press, Milton Keynes

Roush, S. E. (1986) Health professionals as contributors to attitudes towards persons with disabilities. *Physical Therapy*, **66 (10)**, 1551–1554

Sutcliffe, J. (1990) *Adults with Learning Difficulties: Education for Choice and Empowerment*, National Institute of Adult Continuing Education, Leicester

Swain, J. et al. (1993) Introduction. In *Disabling Barriers—Enabling Environments*, (eds J. Swain, V. Finkelstein, S. French and M. Oliver), Sage, London

Understanding Disability Educational Trust (1993) *Understanding Disability* (2nd edn), Understanding Disability Educational Trust, Farnham

UPIAS (1976) *Fundamental Principles of Disability*, Union of the Physically Impaired Against Segregation, London

Wilson, E. D. and Alcorn, D. (1969) Disability simulation and development of attitudes towards the exceptional. *Journal of Special Education*, **3**, 303–307

Wright, B. A. (1980) Developing constructive views of life with a disability. *Rehabilitation Literature*, **41 (11–12)**, 275–279

8

Disabled people and professional practice

Sally French

The relationship between disabled people and health and welfare professionals has never been an easy one, for it is an unequal relationship with the professional holding most of the power. Traditionally professional workers have defined, planned and delivered the services, while disabled people have been passive recipients with little if any opportunity to exercise control. As noted in chapter 1, the definitions disabled people have of the barriers they face, and the appropriate solutions to them, are generally given insufficient weight; this seriously hampers the rehabilitation process, for if there is no consensus little real progress can be made. Gorovitz (1982) points out that if decisions made on behalf of a patient reflect values that are not shared by the patient, his or her autonomy has been overridden in a fundamental way.

The difference in social class between disabled people and professional workers also gives rise to unequal status. Disabled people tend to come from non-professional homes, so they rarely share the same life experiences as the professionals who work with them (Whitehead, 1988). This situation frequently leads to uneasy communication, with disabled people being deferential and inhibited, and professional workers tending to underestimate disabled people's ability to understand complex issues and dilemmas concerning their own lives (Locker, 1982).

What's wrong with professional practice

Disabled people's experiences

It is evident from the writings and recollections of disabled people that professional health and welfare practice can be dehumanizing and abusive. Straughair and Fawcitt (1992) report that the young people with arthritis they interviewed were sometimes accused of being neurotic when their symptoms did not fit into neat diagnostic slots. The relationships they formed with rheumatologists were, however, highly influential; those who had a good relationship were more confident, more ambitious, and less dominated by their symptoms than those who had not.

Lonsdale, reporting on her interviews with disabled women, relates many harmful experiences of hospital treatment and medical care. This particularly concerned doctors who, despite their white coats and other medical trappings, were often perceived by the women as being nothing more than 'groups of anonymous men' (1990: 89). An issue which they repeatedly raised was how frightening they had found their hospital experiences, especially as children. They could recall being asked very personal questions in an insensitive way, of being photographed unclothed, and of being compelled to walk naked in front of medical students.

This 'public stripping', which is now recognized as a form of institutional abuse, was also experienced by Merry, a disabled woman interviewed by Sutherland. She recalls, 'they paraded me up and down on the stage, and the surgeon was saying "who can say what's wrong with this young lady?" ' (1981: 124). Michlene, another disabled woman interviewed by Sutherland, has similar unpleasant recollections. She states:

> My memory is basically of a whole series of experiences of being very coldly and formally mauled around. It's very alienating. It's as if you're a medical specimen. . . . I was never told that I was nice to look at or nice to touch, there was never any feeling of being nice, just of being odd, peculiar. It's horrible. It's taken me years and years to get over it. (1981: 123)

Lonsdale (1990) points out that incidents such as these were recalled by women of all ages and so cannot be dismissed as belonging to 'the bad old days'. Coleridge (1993) believes that the self-image of many disabled people has been damaged by constant involvement with professionals particularly during childhood where play, enjoyment and discovery were replaced by stress, medical examinations and developmental programmes.

Morris interviewed women with spinal cord injuries. Their most common complaint about health and welfare professionals was their lack of concern with emotional issues. One woman said, 'There is no space allowed for us to express our grief. . . . There is often pressure put on us to "cope" and if we fail to live up to the standard demanded of us we are categorised as a "problem" ' (1989: 24). They reported receiving little or no help in coming to terms with sudden paralysis, and often felt compelled to be jolly and play a particular role: as one woman put it, 'the staff expected you to have a smile on your face all the time' (1989: 24). Some women expressed a need for counselling, and said that the only thing that made life bearable for them in hospital was their relationships with other patients. Many of the women believed that the rehabilitation they received was unnecessarily competitive, sport-orientated, and geared towards men. Others thought there was too much emphasis on walking and bladder training. Morris states that the majority of the women:

> found that communication of the vital information about paralysis was poor, that their emotional experience was ignored, that their needs as women were not addressed, and finally that they were given little help in planning for the future. This experience seemed to be as common in the 1980s, as it was during the 1950s, 1960s and 1970s. (1989: 33)

(For further information on gender and disability, the reader is referred to chapter 15.)

Another complaint expressed by disabled people is the emphasis health and welfare professionals place on impairment, while ignoring disability. Maggie, a disabled woman interviewed by Sutherland, explains:

> My criticism of the majority of ear, nose and throat specialists I've had to deal with in the past is that their concern is with my faulty ears, so that if I, as in the early days I did, try to bring up far more important problems than the actual malfunction in my ears, like the effect that it was having on my life, then they would give very abrupt, pat answers which cut the conversation completely dead. (1981: 125)

The issue of professional involvement with disabled people is, however, complex. On the one hand, a narrow focus on impairment ignores important dimensions of the disabled person's experience, but on the other, an expansion of medical involvement, though encouraging a holistic approach, may give health and welfare professionals power to exercise control and make decisions in many areas of the disabled person's life.

Lonsdale (1990) believes that the dismissive, patronizing, punitive and unhelpful attitudes and behaviour which are sometimes displayed towards disabled people by health and welfare professionals, particularly doctors, appear to be due to the following factors: their inability to deal with conditions which are not curable, their unwillingness to admit ignorance or to acknowledge the expertise of disabled people, their desire for a high degree of patient compliance and the lack of practical information they have to offer disabled people. Lonsdale was struck by the warmth and enthusiasm expressed by the women she interviewed for those health and welfare professionals who were prepared to work in partnership with them.

Johnson (1993) interviewed four disabled people who had received physiotherapy. Physiotherapy was largely dismissed as having no importance in their lives. Good experiences were associated with a personal approach, and bad experiences with an impersonal approach where the disabled people felt they were treated as 'passive objects'. Johnson concludes, 'The overwhelming impression was one of disenchantment with physiotherapy . . . its irrelevance to daily life, its failure to ensure understanding and involvement in treatment, and its arrogance in stifling individual autonomy' (1993: 623).

When working with disabled people and allocating resources, it is not unusual for health and welfare professionals to be guided by their own attitudes, values and moral judgements (Stevenson and Parsloe, 1993). Ellis found, for example, that assessments were guided by notions of who were the most deserving of help. She states 'Because self-reliance was positively valued, independent people could be regarded as more deserving of help and, paradoxically, receive more rather than less' (1993: 14). People with knowledge of their entitlements were frequently viewed as 'grabbing', demanding or fussy. Practitioners preferred disabled people who accepted with gratitude what was on offer; those who challenged were described as manipulative, and carers who threatened to withdraw their services were said to be blackmailing. Ellis (1993) found that most disabled people had internalized these views and derived their self-esteem through maintaining or regaining their independence. Those who were prepared to fight received more assistance, but rather than feeling they had scored a victory, their level of stress was increased.

Stevenson and Parsloe stress the importance of self-awareness by those working with disabled people, for example they need to acknowledge over-protectiveness, over anxiety, and 'the hidden satisfaction which they may derive from the benign exercise of power' (1993: 21). However, they also point out that:

> Changing one's attitudes is difficult and not entirely a matter of will. It is more likely to be achieved if the whole climate of the organisation changes and workers can see examples, at all levels, of managers espousing the empowerment, not just of users and carers, but of staff too. (1993: 10)

Stevenson and Parsloe believe that high staff morale contributes to an empowering atmosphere, and that staff must be empowered themselves in order to empower users and carers.

Chinnery (1991) emphasizes the importance of employing disabled professionals, especially at senior and managerial levels, to ensure greater sensitivity to disabled people's requirements. He suggests that the advice of disabled colleagues should be actively sought to discuss and review plans, although this should never be used as an alternative to receiving advice and feedback from those who experience the services first hand. (For further information on disabled health and welfare professionals, the reader is referred to chapter 16.)

The organizational climate

None of these problems are the fault of individual health and welfare professionals, for they are entangled in administrative structures almost as tightly as disabled people themselves. It is important to remember that health and welfare professionals are not completely autonomous; Hugman (1991) explains their role as 'agents of the State' where the State itself, rather than service users, can be viewed as the client.

Marsh and Fisher believe that managers and practitioners are under enormous pressure to take shortcuts and compromise principles, and that 'user-orientated practice requires user-orientated policies' (1992: 38). Ellis (1993) notes that advocating for a client can put practitioners into conflict with employers, and Stevenson and Parsloe contend that, 'without a new culture there will be severe limitations on what workers can do' (1993: 9). Chinnery states:

> Individual workers may well act in non-disabling ways, but the structure of services which reaches far beyond that which is visible to disabled users, militates actively and very effectively against individual efforts to promote a helpful, non-disabling, client orientated service. (1990a: 53)

The organizational context and culture should not, however, be used as an excuse for doing nothing, Stevenson and Parsloe (1993) found many examples of workers trying to empower clients in the face of organizational opposition. They found workers creating 'islands' of empowerment over matters in which they had some influence, and believe that giving disabled people choice concerns small as well as large issues.

Professional dominance and power

A central theme throughout this book has been the ways in which the physical and social environment disables people with impairments. The education and role of health and welfare professionals, however, leads them to ignore this fact. Brechin and Liddiard state 'Clinical work has traditionally occurred on the basis of individual referral, and assessment procedures have evolved around the assumption that in the individual lies the problem and the solution' (1981: 40).

Barnes is harsh in his judgement of rehabilitation services believing them to be 'highly discriminatory' and 'a major disservice to disabled people' (1991: 132). He states, 'with the removal of the economic and social barriers which confront disabled people, the need for rehabilitation in its present form would be greatly reduced or eliminated altogether' (1991: 132). He recognizes that the role of health and welfare professionals is to help disabled people to cope with an impossibly difficult environment, a process which, he believes, would not be tolerated if practised on any other section of society. Merry, a disabled woman interviewed by Sutherland, agrees; she states, 'The whole professional intervention is a waste of time unless they start making a society which is going to be accessible to all of us, which treats us all with dignity and humanity' (1981: 131).

Focusing on impairment is not, however, wrong; most people would agree, for example, that it is sensible to strengthen muscles, move joints and assist a person's balance following a spinal cord injury. Treatment may also be justified in terms of the way society is structured at the present time. This does, however, give rise to a difficult dilemma, for concentrating on the impairment, rather than on social and physical barriers, tends to maintain the status quo. Biklen (1988) contends that clinical judgements cannot be viewed apart from the political context.

Community and health provision is largely 'provider led' rather than 'consumer led'. As Barton states: 'The overwhelming activities and noise with regard to both policy and practice have emanated from professionals. It is professional values and objectives which have defined needs and practice' (1993: 255). This is not because disabled people have nothing to say, but because they have been given little opportunity to speak

Policies and services tend to be framed in terms of people's per-ceived deficits, rather than their capabilities, and needs are adapted to match available provision. Ellis (1993) believes that this leads practitioners to make stereotyped responses to disabled people's needs, drawing on the limited range of provision and services avail-able, and with which they are familiar. Thus assessment is used as a way of managing demand and may, in itself, be rationed (Ellis, 1993). With no direct purchasing power disabled people are forced to rely on the 'menu' of services provided. Ellis (1993) believes that any rationing of services should be 'up front' so that disabled people can challenge it.

Rationing and 'provider-led' services should not be blamed en-tirely on lack of resources, however. Stevenson and Parsloe make the point that 'Innovation is not necessarily associated with periods of expansion' (1993: 37), and Ellis contends that stereotyped responses to the needs of disabled people 'resulted as much from a failure of imagination as a shortage of resources' (1993: 19).

Services are defined by health and welfare professionals, and are based around pre-existing skills, techniques and facilities which are only available at specific times. Professional dominance can be seen in assessment procedures where, for example, the therapist's or nurse's observations may be viewed as objective whereas the patient's perceptions are viewed as subjective (Coates and King, 1982), and where pseudo-scientific language serves to mystify and confuse the patient or client (Grieve, 1988; French, 1991; Hugman, 1991). Because of the specialization of the various professional groups, definitions of need tend to be narrow, their scope being dictated by specialized knowledge and interests (Ellis, 1993). The needs of disabled people, on the other hand, tend to be multifaceted. As Marsh and Fisher point out:

> If the process of assessment becomes one of professional discovery of 'need', rather than a negotiation of problems, then users tend to feel hemmed in by the definitions used to describe their circumstances and trapped by the choices they are faced with. (1992: 5O)

Professionals usually receive above average pay, high status, and autonomy in their work. They have the power to control the encounter with their patients or clients; setting the agenda, managing time to suit their own schedules, defining problems and the appropriate solutions to them and making all the decisions. Oliver (1990) contends that this translates political problems into technical and technological problems. He goes on to explain that the language professionals use, relating to both problems and solutions, makes the evaluation of services extremely difficult for disabled people. This removes disability from the realm of normality and has the potential for producing feelings of inadequacy and inertia in non-medical members of society, as well as disabled people themselves. The power of the professions is compounded by the ways in which they collaborate with each other; disabled people, in contrast, have had little opportunity, until recent times, to come together in this way.

Because disability has been medicalized, disabled people often find they are compelled to go through a medical professional, or a bureaucratic agency, to get a service they require or a piece of equipment they need. Professional dominance can thus render services for disabled people limited, inconvenient, inefficient and frustrating; community-care policies have done little to improve this situation. Oliver (1990) refers to professionals as the 'gatekeepers' of scarce resources, a situation which leaves disabled people with little choice but to accept what is on offer. Professional dominance and control is a vital issue for disabled people because health and welfare professionals frequently involve themselves, not only in medical matters, but in many areas of disabled people's lives, such as their education, employment and accommodation. Stevenson and Parsloe (1993) believe that the philosophy of service should change from that of problem solving to that of user and carer empowerment.

The medicalization of everyday life has been conceptualized by many sociologists, for example Irving (1972), Illich (1976) and Conrad (1979), as a form of social control. The labelling of political dissidents as mentally ill is an obvious example of this. Disability is particularly susceptible to the process of medicalization because of the physical nature of impairment, and the important contribution that medicine can sometimes make. Illich (1976), a prominent critic of medical practice, believes that the permeation of medicine into people's lives diminishes their autonomy, increases their dependency and fosters the false impression that most problems can be solved by medicine. This is not to say that the difficulties disabled people may face cannot be viewed in medical terms, but to argue that within an individualistic approach that is the *only* way they are viewed (Shakespeare, 1993).

Coleridge (1993) agrees that the emphasis on rehabilitation perpetuates the idea that disabled people must be taken care of, normalized, and treated as perpetual patients. Hurst (1987) and Finkelstein (1990) point out that despite severe poverty, organizations of disabled people find it easier to flourish in developing countries than developed countries, partly because of their lack of bureaucratic and professional structure. Ways must be found to promote professional services without diminishing the capacity of disabled people to confront, in political terms, the issues which affect their lives.

Oliver points out that medical need is often viewed as more important than other needs. He states:

> medical need still predominates over educational need; disabled children still have operations (necessary and unnecessary) at times which fit in with the schedule of surgeons and hospitals rather than educational programmes, children are still taken out of classes for doctor's appointments or physiotherapy, and the school nurse is still a more influential figure than the teachers. (1990: 92)

Similarly, Mason and Rieser state:

> For young people the disadvantages of medical treatment need to be weighed against the possible advantages. Children are not usually asked if they want speech therapy, physiotherapy, orthopaedic surgery, hospitalisation, drugs, or cumbersome and ugly 'aids and appliances'. We are not asked if we want to be put on daily regimes or programmes which use hours of precious play-time. All these things are just imposed on us with the assumption that we share our parents' or therapists' desire for us to be more 'normal' at all costs. We are not even consulted as adults as to whether we think those things had been necessary or useful. (1992: 82)

It is important to remember that health and well-being are frequently tied to social, economic and political factors (Smith and Jacobson, 1988), and that medical problems are rarely of paramount importance in disabled people's lives (British Psychological Society,

1989). Frazer reports that at a forum of over one hundred disabled people, organized by a health district, 'not one individual mentioned any further need for doctors or medical support' (1988: 6). (For a detailed account of power in the caring professions, the reader is referred to Hugman, 1991.)

Improving professional practice

To achieve relevant and high quality services for disabled people, there need to be changes in both education and practice. It is important that health and welfare professionals receive high quality disability equality training, that they understand the meaning of disability as disabled people define it, that they are informed about the important role disabled people have played in the development of services, and that they present information to disabled people in accessible formats. This, however, is not enough. To be truly effective health and welfare professionals must relinquish their power and control and work closely with disabled people under their direction. As Munro and Elder-Woodward state, 'The challenge for workers at all levels of community care is to make sure that the service user is in control of his own lifestyle *and* in control of the services surrounding him which are designed to support that lifestyle' (1992: 41).

Butterworth (1988), talking of community nurses, believes that they should become politically aware and at the forefront of social action. He notes that few nurse education programmes demonstrate a commitment to political awareness or political involvement. Ellis (1993) believes that the most effective way of empowering disabled people is to bring them together in order that they may share their experiences.

Marsh and Fisher (1992) give many suggestions for the improvement of services which include:

- Finding ways of integrating unique user characteristics into assessment procedures.
- Negotiating with users of services as the primary means of identifying problems and solutions.
- Ensuring there is a feedback channel for the views of users.
- Having an organizational ethos of accountability to users, and ensuring that practitioners and managers are able to view services from the users' perspective.

Finkelstein (1991) believes that the central focus of disability services should take place in Centres for Integrated Living, which are controlled by disabled people themselves (see chapter 6), and that disability services should be placed in the Department of the Environment, rather than the Department of Health. He states: 'workers in rehabilitation services should see themselves as a resource, to be tapped by disabled clients, rather than as professionals trained to make highly specialised assessments of what is appropriate for individual disabled people' (1991: 36). Collaboration among professionals and other service providers from various disciplines, with disabled people themselves, would widen perspectives and help to develop new ideas and practices. For example, architects, social workers, occupational therapists and disabled people could join forces to effect imaginative changes in housing policy and design; Wilson (1990) explains, for example, how the Department of Health has funded an occupational therapist to work closely with housing agencies. Collaboration in research is also needed to avoid the perpetuation of a narrow medical view of disability.

Professional practice—the place of counselling

It is perhaps surprising, given that many disabled people reject the notion that disability is an internal state of body or mind, that many express a need for counselling. It has been seen, however, that becoming disabled can, for some people at least, be a psychologically devastating experience (see chapter 2). Constantly confronting barriers, hostile attitudes and discriminatory practices can also have adverse psychological effects, sometimes leading disabled people to become unduly shy and passive. Nearly a quarter of the blind and partially-sighted people surveyed by the visual impairment group (Lomas, 1993), for example, expressed a need for counselling, and counselling is a major service offered by Centres of Integrated Living (see chapter 6).

Chinnery (1990b) believes that disabled people often receive a hostile or over-emotional response if they so much as mention their disability, and that they are rewarded for behaving in a passive, compliant way and punished for becoming angry or assertive. Safilios-Rothschild (1970) notes that the label 'unmotivated' is given to patients when they refuse to perform the prescribed therapeutic activities, or when they do not agree with the rehabilitation worker's definition of the problem and the appropriate solutions. As choice regarding services is usually non-existent, disabled people are under extreme pressure to 'stay on the right side' of health and welfare professionals, resulting in further feelings of inhibition. Frazer (1988), reporting on a forum run by a health district to discover what disabled people want, states 'The most noticeable phenomenon of the day was the remarkable anger expressed by the majority of the participants'.

But then, in apparent disapproval, he goes on to say 'It was perhaps fortuitous that each group was led by a psychologist who could re-direct the anger into a more positive form of expression' (1988: 6). Traits which are labelled 'bad' are, however, often the ones which are needed by disabled people to prosper within a disabling society. Chinnery (1990b) believes that disabled people's anger is constructive and must be understood, valued and actively rewarded.

Counselling is an area where professional workers may be well placed, with appropriate training, to assist disabled people (Chinnery, 1990b). There are a wide variety of counselling approaches which can be adopted (see Thomson, 1992). Lenny (1993) rejects behavioural approaches for use with disabled people, because they assume the problems encountered arise from within the individual, rather than from within society. She advocates client-centred approaches as they encourage people to explore and express their own thoughts, feelings and desires without intervention or evaluation by the counsellor.

Behavioural approaches should not be disregarded completely, however. Assertiveness training, for example, is a behavioural approach where disabled people may be encouraged to role play difficult situations, such as confronting a colleague who is behaving in a patronizing way at work. Cognitive counselling may also be useful. In this approach, damaging thinking patterns, where, for example, disabled people are telling themselves they are unattractive or unintelligent, are confronted and assistance given in replacing them with more positive thoughts. This approach may help some disabled people who, through their life experiences, have developed low self-esteem and self-confidence. These counselling methods may encourage disabled people to act on their own behalf by expressing their feelings, desires and needs in a self-assured and confident way.

In order to counsel disabled people effectively it is vital that health and welfare professionals have a thorough understanding of disability. Finkelstein (1990) believes that none of the existing service approaches to disability were set up on the basis of a thorough understanding of it, and that the practice of health and welfare professionals has not generated an in-depth analysis of the meaning of disability. Similarly Stevens states:

> If effective user-led services are to be developed, it is important for non-disabled practitioners to develop an understanding of disability from disabled people's point of view. They are not likely to develop this simply through reflective practice as their own experience of disability and those of the practitioners around them is likely to have come through negative cultural stereotypes which emphasise tragic loss and dependency. (1993: 27)

The need for a thorough understanding of disability can be illustrated by considering genetic counselling and abortion. Many

people view genetic counselling as a helpful way of preventing disabled children from being born. Disabled people, in contrast, may find
such a view highly offensive. Reynolds states:

> What is unreasonable to me is the 'moral' pressures which I believe are
> brought to bear to persuade the mother to have an abortion for the sake
> of the child. . . . Just because someone else cannot imagine how I can
> put up with living with my disability does not mean that I should never
> have been born. It simply means that they have a limited imagination.
> (1990: 8)

Mason (1992) believes that genetic counselling should be offered, but
not in a way which implies that having a disabled baby is wrong or
bad. Reynolds (1990) and Morris (1991) have criticized the fact that
the legal time limit for the abortion of 'seriously handicapped' foetuses is longer than that for all other foetuses.

Sutherland (1981) questions the wisdom of genetic counselling,
recalling the little publicized fact that 100,000 disabled people were
exterminated in Nazi Germany. Similarly Morris states:

> The arguments about whether disabled people's lives are worth living,
> and whether the medical profession should enable us to be 'released
> from misery' are as threatening today as they were in the Germany of
> the 1930s and early 1940s. We need to question fundamentally the
> assumption that to be disabled, to be different, means that life is not
> worth living. (1991: 58)

(For further information on genetic counselling and abortion in relation to disability, the reader is referred to Morris, 1991.)

Conclusion

Over the last twenty years disabled people have become increasingly
organized and politically active; Centres for Integrated Living, coalitions of disabled people and international disability organizations, all
controlled by disabled people themselves, now flourish. There are
radio and television programmes promoting the views of disabled
people, and an increasing number of conferences, courses, journals
and books on disability issues, organized and produced by disabled
academics. All of this amounts to a disability movement as disabled
people press for control in decision-making and for their perspectives
and rights to be acknowledged and acted upon. Though still young,
the movement has brought about considerable change in attitudes
and practices (see chapter 6).

Health and welfare professionals understandably tend to find these
developments threatening, as their status, power, roles and even their
jobs no longer seem secure. It has to be admitted that there are some

disabled people who, disillusioned with the treatment they have received in the past, reject any professional involvement in the new services they are developing. However, many believe that partnership and collaboration with professional workers is important, and professionals are already assisting disabled people in developing services appropriate to their needs as they define them. Professionals in such a situation serve as a resource to disabled people as they strive to reach their own goals. They do not attempt to dominate, to take control or to *manage* disabled people, but rather to act as supportive enablers, actively sharing their expertise and knowledge while recognizing the expertise of disabled people and learning from them (see chapter 18).

Such a change of relationship requires a radical shift in the balance of power, making the traditional professional role untenable. This does not mean that the professional worker is no longer needed or valued, but rather that new, perhaps more rewarding, roles must be created. Munro and Elder-Woodward believe that 'It is only when staff look upon service users as equals, and treat them with the respect that an equal deserves, that they develop their own self worth' (1992: 30). (For detailed advice on user participation and the evaluation of services, readers are referred to Fiedler, 1991, Fiedler and Twitchin, 1992; Marsh and Fisher, 1992; Ellis, 1993 and Stevenson and Parsloe, 1993.)

Health and welfare professionals are in a difficult position in effecting change for to do so may involve criticizing their managers, their colleagues, the philosophy and practice of their places of employment and their professional education. In addition individual professional workers rarely have control of resources, which are so often at the root of service delivery decisions and practice. Health and welfare professionals are thus locked into work structures which are difficult to challenge or change, a situation which frequently leads to compromises not necessarily reflecting the health or welfare professionals' ideas or intentions. The changes needed are thus not only administrative and social, but also political.

Although few nurses or therapists have the power or resources to bring about large changes of policy, it is wrong to conclude that nothing can be achieved by the individual. Small changes, for example giving disabled people more choice regarding their treatment, or responding to their views during assessment, can be very important and sometimes fuel more radical changes of policy. For meaningful change to take place, however, it must be done on disabled people's terms.

Many innovations by disabled people, which could provide excellent models of practice, have been ignored by service providers. Chinnery believes that not to act on information coming from disabled people is morally indefensible as well as damaging to service providers themselves. He asks:

> can we afford to avoid the fact that services to disabled people are inadequate, poorly focused, disabling and discriminatory? The 'bottom line' is that users of our services will most certainly be very unhappy if these matters are not tackled. Can the caring services afford to risk this unpopularity amongst such a large and increasingly vocal proportion of the population? (1990a: 53)

Change is often stressful which makes it easy for service providers to avoid it and maintain the status quo, yet although changes in practice will undoubtedly involve some personal and professional costs, both parties are likely to experience considerable personal growth and satisfaction if action can be initiated and change can be faced.

References

Barnes, C. (1991) *Disabled People in Britain and Discrimination*, Hurst & Company, London

Barton, L. (1993) The struggle for citizenship: the case of disabled people. *Disability, Handicap and Society*, **8 (3)**, 235–248

Biklen, D. (1988) The myth of clinical judgement. *Journal of Social Issues*, **4 (1)**, 127–140

Brechin, A. and Liddiard, P. (1981) *Look at it This Way—New Perspectives in Rehabilitation*, Hodder & Stoughton, Sevenoaks

British Psychological Society (1989) *Psychology and Physical Disability in the National Health Service*. Report of the Professional Affairs Board of The British Psychological Society, Leicester

Butterworth, T. (1988) Political awareness. *Community*, December, 20–21

Chinnery, B. (1990a) Disabled people get the message: non-verbal clues to the nature of social work. *Practice*, **4 (1)**, 49–55

Chinnery, B. (1990b) The process of being disabled. *Practice*, **4 (1)**, 43–48

Chinnery, B. (1991) Equal opportunities for disabled people in the caring professions: window dressing or commitment? *Disability, Handicap and Society*, **6 (3)**, 253–258

Coates, H. and King, A. (1982) *The Patient Assessment*, Churchill Livingstone, Edinburgh

Coleridge, P. (1993) *Disability, Liberation and Empowerment*, Oxfam, Oxford

Conrad, P. (1979) Types of medical social control. *Sociology of Health and Illness*, **1 (1)**, 1–11

Ellis, K. (1993) *Squaring the Circle: User and Carer Participation in Needs Assessment*, Joseph Rowntree Foundation, London

Fiedler, B. (1991) Tracking success: testing services for people with severe physical and sensory disabilities. *Living Options in Practice*, Project paper 2, The Prince of Wales Advisory Group on Disability and the King's Fund Centre, London

Fiedler, B. and Twitchin, D. (1992) Achieving user participation: planning services for people with severe physical and sensory disabilities. *Living Options in Practice*, Project Paper 3. The Prince of Wales Advisory Group on Disability and the King's Fund Centre, London

Finkelstein, V. (1990) Services for clients or clients for services? Paper given at the annual course of the North Regional Association of the Blind. 18 October

Finkelstein, V. (1991) Disability: an administrative challenge? In *Social Work, Disabled People and Disabling Environments*, (ed. M. Oliver), Jessica Kingsley, London

Frazer, F. (1988) Letting off steam. *Therapy Weekly*, **15 (23)**, 6

French, S. (1991) Setting a record straight. *Therapy Weekly*, **18 (1)**, 4

Gorovitz, S. (1982) *Doctors' Dilemmas: Moral Conflict and Medical Care*, Oxford University Press, Oxford

Grieve, G. P. (1988) Clinical examination and the SOAP mnemonic. *Physiotherapy*, **74 (2)**, 97

Hugman, R. (1991) *Power in Caring Professions*, Macmillan, London

Hurst, R. (1987) A voice to be reckoned with. *Disability Now*, February, 6

Illich, I. (1976) *Limits to Medicine*, Penguin Books, Harmondsworth

Irving, K. (1972) Medicine as an institution of social control. *Social Review*, **20**, 487–503

Johnson, R. (1993) 'Attitudes don't just hang in the air' . . . disabled people's perceptions of physiotherapists. *Physiotherapy*, **79 (9)**, 619–626

Lenny, J. (1993) Do disabled people need counselling? In *Disabling Barriers—Enabling Environments*, (eds J. Swain, V. Finkelstein, S. French and M. Oliver), Sage, London

Locker, D. (1982) Communication in medical practice. In *Sociology as Applied to Medicine*, (D. L. Patrick and G. Scambler), Bailliere-Tindall, London

Lomas, G. (1993) *A New Deal for Blind and Partially Sighted People*, report of a working party set up by the visual handicap group, Royal National Institute for the Blind, London

Lonsdale, S. (1990) *Women and Disability*, Macmillan, London

Marsh, P. and Fisher, M. (1992) *Good Intentions: Developing Partnership in Social Services*, Joseph Rowntree Foundation, London

Mason, M. (1992) Sexuality and disability. In *Disability Equality in the*

Classroom: A Human Rights Issue, (2nd edn), (eds R. Rieser and M. Mason), Disability Equality in Education, London

Mason, M. and Rieser, R. (1992) The limits of medicine. In *Disability Equality in the Classroom: A Human Rights Issue*, (2nd edn), (eds R. Rieser and M. Mason), Disability Equality in Education, London

Morris, J. (1989) *Able Lives*, The Women's Press, London

Morris, J. (1991) *Pride Against Prejudice*, The Women's Press, London

Munro, K. and Elder-Woodward, J. (1992) *Independent Living*, Churchill Livingstone, Edinburgh

Oliver, M. (1990) *The Politics of Disablement*, Macmillan, London

Reynolds, A. (1990) Is it good to avoid awkward choices? *Disability Now*, June, 8

Safilios-Rothschild, C. (1970) *The Sociology and Social Psychology of Disability and Rehabilitation*, Random House, New York

Shakespeare, T. (1993) Disabled people's self-organisation: a new social movement? *Disability, Handicap and Society*, **8 (3)**, 249–264

Smith, A. and Jacobson, B. (1988) *The Nation's Health*, King's Fund Publishing Office, London

Stevens, A. (1993) Communicating with users: learning a user led perspective through reflective practice. In *Back from the Wellhouse: Discussion Papers on Sensory Impairment and Training in Community Care*, (ed. A. Stevens), Central Council for Education and Training in Social Work, London

Stevenson, O. and Parsloe, P. (1993) *Community Care and Empowerment*, Joseph Rowntree Foundation, London

Straughair, S. and Fawcitt, S. (1992) *The Road Towards Independence: The Experiences of Young People with Arthritis in the 1990s*, Arthritis Care, London

Sutherland, A. T. (1981) *Disabled We Stand*, Souvenir Press, London

Thomson, D. J. (1992) Counselling. In *Physiotherapy: A Psychosocial Approach*, (ed. S. French), Butterworth-Heinemann, Oxford

Whitehead, M. (1988) *Inequalities in Health: The Health Divide*, Penguin Books, Harmondsworth

Wilson, P. (1990) Going home. *Therapy Weekly*, **17 (18)**, 10

9

Institutional and community living

Sally French

Before discussing institutional and community living, it is necessary to explore what is meant by 'institution' and 'community'.

Institution

The term 'institution' has various meanings, for example the family and marriage are institutions, as is any repeated or continuous practice maintained by social norms. In the present context, 'institution' refers to 'an organization or establishment founded for a specific purpose' (McLeod, (1986: 441)). Institutions are very varied, ranging from those which are well integrated within society to those which are totally isolated. The latter are referred to as 'total' or 'closed' institutions. They are characterized by rigid routines with little or no attention being paid to individual needs. Daily activities such as working, eating, sleeping and exercise are carried out in groups within the same environment, and the many rules and regulations exist more for the benefit of the staff than the residents. According to Humphries and Gordon (1992) the underlying purpose of closed institutions is to crush people's individual personalities in order to ensure conformity. Goffman, in his famous book *Asylums*, describes a total institution as 'a place of residence and work where a large number of like situated individuals, cut off from the wider society for an appreciable period of time, together lead an enclosed, formally administered round of life' (1961: 11).

The incarceration of people considered to be deviant became commonplace in the nineteenth century and expanded rapidly in the first half of the twentieth century. Since then there has been an overall decline, although Hunt (1992) points out the marked growth of segregated facilities for disabled people in the 1960s and 1970s; the residents of Cheshire homes, for example, rose from 457 in 1961 to 1402 in 1970 (Hunt, 1992: 26). Finkelstein remarks on the many honours which have been showered on non-disabled people, by other non-disabled people, for removing disabled people from mainstream society. He states:

> There is a singular lack of awareness that there may be something profoundly undemocratic about able-bodied people supporting the systematic removal of disabled people from their communities, that it is only able-bodied people who write glowingly about each other for having done this to disabled people, and that it is able-bodied people who give themselves awards for this contribution to the isolation of disabled people from the mainstream of life. (1991: 19)

Conditions labelled 'mental handicap' and 'mental illness' were 'medicalized' and the institutions where such people were detained adopted strict hospital rules and routines, often in the absence of any meaningful treatment; indeed the health needs of the 'patients' were frequently neglected (Oswin, 1978). It was extremely common to incarcerate physically-disabled people, including children, in these institutions too. It was not until the 1960s that any serious challenge to these practices was made. This followed several damning theoretical analyses of total institutions by sociologists such as Goffman (1961) and Townsend (1962), and later the uncovering of considerable abuse and cruelty. At the same time people such as Szasz (1961) and Laing (1967) were attacking the very concept of insanity, and advances in drug therapy made it more feasible to discharge people with schizophrenia and depressive illness from hospital; the growing civil rights movement may also have had an effect. Along with these changes, the large institutions were becoming difficult to staff and maintain, and were increasingly recognized as expensive, outdated and stigmatizing. However, government policy explicitly advocating 'community care' did not gain momentum until the 1980s.

In contrast to total institutions, there are those which attempt to integrate into society. They are generally small and well staffed with residents having more autonomy over their lives, as well as opportunities for involvement in policy making. This type of institution has become more common as total institutions have declined.

Precisely when an 'institution' should be regarded as a 'community home' or part of 'the community' is impossible to say, but it certainly has less to do with size than the style of management, the attitudes and behaviour of staff and the availability of resources. An institutionalized atmosphere can be created in a small group home, or even a family, just as a homely atmosphere can be created in a large institution, albeit with difficulty. Davidson is of the opinion that relationships in the community may be 'almost as debilitatingly dependent and institutional as any relationship in a long-stay hospital' (1987: 180), and Morris (1993) makes the point that, rather than being dismantled, institutions can be dispersed within the community. Holmes and Johnson (1988) give a detailed account of the deprived lives of old people living in private nursing homes, many of which are very small.

One of the major criticisms of institutions is their geographical isolation. This creates problems for residents who want to socialize outside the institution and for staff who are encouraging them to do so. It makes regular visiting by families and friends more difficult and inhibits other people from becoming involved. It is also one of the factors giving rise to staffing problems. This physical isolation was sometimes planned, as in the case of psychiatric hospitals built in the nineteenth century, and sometimes a matter of convenience. Following the 1944 Education Act, for example, many large, isolated houses in the countryside were used as special residential schools, simply because they were available. To compound this situation, many people are socially isolated before entering institutions and any contacts and relationships they have tend to be unstable. This was recognized in the Warnock Report of 1978 with regard to children in special residential schools.

This social and geographical isolation, together with the powerlessness of the residents, can lead to considerable neglect and abuse which often remains undiscovered and unchallenged (Westcott, 1991; Humphries and Gordon, 1992; French, 1992; Marchant and Page, 1992; Westcott, 1993). Potts and Fido (1991), in their interviews with people detained in mental-handicap hospitals, give graphic evidence of abuse perpetrated by professional staff; the inmates were totally controlled by the system while at the same time suffering severe neglect.

It is generally believed that abuse is less likely to occur in community settings as 'the community' provides its own watchdog, but some people have argued that abuse is more likely in the community because systematic inspection is so difficult. Morris (1993b), in her study of independent living, found that most of the disabled people she interviewed could recall instances where helpers were patronizing and verbally or physically abusive. One of the reasons that abuse of disabled people, both inside and outside institutions, remains uncovered, is that many people have difficulty believing it exists, whereas in reality, disabled people appear to be at greater risk from abuse than others (Westcott, 1993). (For further information on the abuse of disabled people, the reader is referred to chapter 14.)

Because of the lack of facilities to overcome physical and social barriers, as well as their social isolation, the residents of institutions are often unduly dependent on staff for their social and emotional, as well as their physical, needs. Thus any opposition to the treatment they receive may result in adverse labelling, which in turn may lead to greater isolation or harsher treatment. In this situation it is impossible for residents to complain without making themselves more vulnerable. Talking of disabled children in special schools during the first half of the twentieth century, Humphries and Gordon state that 'The opportunity for children to resist such a harsh system of control and punishment was extremely limited. They were under immense psychological pressure to obey the rules at all times' (1992: 92). Morris (1993a) also found that disabled people living in institutions found it difficult to complain.

Although many staff working in institutions do their utmost for the welfare of the residents, often against tremendous odds, institutions sometimes attract inadequate people who find it difficult to cope in mainstream society themselves. Vaizey (1959) believes that people attracted to working in institutions are inadequate, unfulfilled, insecure and authoritarian, with a lust for power and control; over the years they become increasingly institutionalized themselves. Such people are often untrained, poorly educated and under paid. They frequently develop low expectations of the residents in their charge and a hostile attitude to outsiders. The influence of the environment on the behaviour of staff must not, however, be underestimated. The staff of institutions are often working in a depressing and stressful environment with inadequate resources or support. Even well-meaning staff may have inappropriate attitudes and behaviour patterns, for example they may have low expectations of disabled people's abilities.

Staff who have direct contact with disabled residents are usually at the bottom of an authoritarian hierarchy where they are virtually forced to behave in the way that they do (Orford, 1980). Sedgwick believes that nurses 'frequently find themselves up against sets of rules and social mores which do not seem to have changed since the last century' (1989: 30). Oswin (1978) found that young nurses working with children with learning difficulties were discouraged, against their better judgement, from mothering them. In time the attitudes and behaviour of staff may become custodial and punitive in order to conform and reduce psychological conflict which tends to occur if a person's behaviour and attitudes are at variance. Despite the harshness of the environment, some staff do, however, manage to maintain their humanity (Potts and Fido, 1991).

The behaviour of disabled people may also be affected by the environment. People have a tendency to live up to what others expect of them, a process known as the 'self-fulfilling prophecy'. Disabled people in institutions may emulate the expectations of the staff, reinforcing erroneous stereotypes and prejudices which justify the institution's existence. The social, emotional and intellectual deprivation which can result from institutional living may also lead disabled people to become institutionalized. People with learning difficulties and multiple impairments may, in particular, suffer from the ill-effects of a barren environment as they may be unable to create their own stimulation; thus psychological problems can be caused by the system of care itself. Ford (1987) explains that after years of incarceration residents need considerable assistance in coping successfully with life in mainstream society. Thus the presence of institutions tends to confirm their need and inhibit the adoption of other, more creative, approaches.

The lack of flexibility within some institutions hinders independence as everything must be done by a certain time and in a specific way. Wilkinson (1987) notes how the independence of mentally ill people is reduced by nurses who do too much for them, and Cooke (1987) believes that the independence of old people in geriatric wards is sometimes restricted to the extent of infringing their civil liberties. Many severely disabled people, who leave institutions for a life in the community, are surprised at how much they are able to achieve (Davis, 1981; Shearer, 1982). Even institutions which express a specific aim to encourage independence may in reality be restrictive because any attempt to enhance self-sufficiency is offset by institutional rules and regulations.

The institutionalization of disabled people and their removal from mainstream society has the tendency to increase the stigma attached to their impairments and to worsen the fears and prejudices of the general public. The education of the public is often put forward as a major reason for the closure of institutions and the integration of disabled people in 'the community'. It is believed that people will never accept difference in their fellow citizens unless they are fully informed and have contact with them on an equal basis from an early age. Whether this acceptance actually occurs, however, is open to question. With regard to deaf children Meadow (1980) and Ladd (1990) are very sceptical. The attitudes and feelings of disabled children attending special and mainstream schools are also very mixed (Booth and Statham, 1982; Madge and Fassam, 1982; Wade and Moore, 1993).

Some people believe it is immoral to subject disabled people to an unsatisfactory community situation just to serve the function of educating the public, though disabled people would obviously stand to gain eventually if attitudes and behaviour towards them became more positive. The knowledge and attitudes of the general public towards people living in institutions tend to be poor (McConkey, 1987); this obviously mitigates against a happy and successful 'community' experience, at least in the short-term. Davidson (1987) believes that because of the attitudes of society and the pressure this puts on people who do not match society's expectations and standards, there may, in some circumstances and for some individuals, be a need for well-run asylums. Davidson (1987) believes that even if the inadequacy of institutional living is accepted, it can still be inhumane to eject people into 'the community' when they have known no other home for many years.

An infrequently expressed view is that people with impairments may prefer to live with those who are similarly affected. Indeed the emphasis on integration may disguise a deep-rooted negativism, for there is an implicit assumption that disabled people will be happier and more fulfilled in the 'normal' community, that they prefer the lifestyle and company of those without disability, and that they wish to be as 'normal' as possible. There is rarely any reference to the frustrations and disadvantages that integration and striving for independence and 'normality' may create, or the benefits derived from being with other disabled people in terms of empathy, friendship and the wealth of knowledge to be shared.

Harrison (1987) gives many examples of disabled people living in institutions who prefer the lifestyle to that of more independent living. Morris (1993) found that some disabled people she interviewed viewed residential care as giving them freedom because of the constant availability of staff, while others saw it as a stepping stone to independence from the family home. It is likely, however, that these views were expressed in the light of inadequate community services and facilities.

Tully (1986) makes many suggestions for improving institutional life for disabled people. He believes that the principle of 'the least restrictive alternative' should operate at all times. This means that the environment must present the smallest possible restraint and disruption to the disabled person's well-being and preferred lifestyle. He believes that residents should be fully involved in decision making, including any concerning their own treatment and assessment, and that any records which are kept should be fully accessible to residents and reflect their own perspectives. Residents should not be prevented from taking risks and should be provided with sufficient privacy for relationships to develop. Every attempt should be made to integrate fully the institution with the community, according to the wishes of the residents.

The function of institutions

There are various views regarding the major functions of institutions. Professional rhetoric is usually in terms of 'treatment' and helping residents to reach their full potential, but others believe that they exist in order to enable mainstream society to run smoothly. Certainly many concerns have been expressed about the effects on non-disabled people of closing institutions and integrating disabled people within society.

Institutions may also have the function of socializing disabled people to play a specific role. Scott (1969) gives a graphic account of rehabilitation centres for newly visually-impaired people, where they are taught the behaviour and attitudes thought necessary to play the role of 'blind person'. The underlying philosophy of the majority of institutions is that disability is contained within the individual rather than within society, it is therefore viewed as a problem for the individual to 'overcome'. The staff of institutions are rarely in the business of encouraging people to challenge disabling physical and social barriers and attitudes which stand in their way. (For further information on the disabled role, the reader is referred to chapter 4.)

The initial encounter with the service provider may occur at a time when the disabled person is particularly vulnerable, either physically or psychologically. At a time such as this disabled people may, understandably, be uncritical and unusually trusting, only later realizing that measures to solve the difficulties they are experiencing have been instigated and may be inappropriate. A further problem is that there is generally a lack of rehabilitation options which forces disabled people to accept whatever is on offer. As Davis puts it, 'the choice available to us amounts to little more than Hobson's choice' (1993: 198).

One of the justifications for the existence of institutions is that scarce and expensive resources, in terms of equipment and staff expertise, can be pooled. However, many people believe that such resources and services can and should be available within the community and that institutions should not be justified on these grounds. It is easy to overestimate the importance of resources; the attitudes of ordinary people and their willingness to consult with and learn from those they wish to assist, are just as important. It is often the case that a reallocation of resources, rather than more resources, is all that is needed.

Without doubt one of the factors which has hindered the closure of institutions, is the vested interests of the staff who work in them. If they close staff will have to work in a different way, in new surroundings, or may lose their jobs altogether. Professionals have defined and maintained institutions according to their own perspectives and interests, often viewing disabled people as less like others than they really are. They may welcome neither closure nor a shift to 'the community' (Ryan and Thomas, 1987). Professionals are part of the institutional environment and it is therefore not always in their own interests to question that environment too closely (McConkey, 1987). Illich (1976) and many others have argued that practices claimed by professionals to benefit clients often serve their own interests more.

The large institutions have been inherited from a time when ideas about illness, disability and deviance were different from those held today (Mittler, 1979). People with learning difficulties, for example, were thought to be dangerous, promiscuous, and a threat to society. No large and complex social system is easy to dismantle and will frequently persist even though those working within it, as well as the wider society, view it as divisive or have ceased to believe in its value. In order to reduce the psychological conflict this creates, people tend to find justifications for the existence and continuance of institutions which often have little in common with the original philosophy, or the reality of how they came to be.

Community

Abercrombie et al. believe the concept of 'community' is 'one of the most elusive and vague within sociology' and that it is now 'without specific meaning' (1988: 44). Richman refers to the concept as one of 'infinite elasticity' (1987: 185). The notion of 'community' can refer to a group of people within a given geographical area, a collection of people living within a particular social structure or a psychological entity; for example, we talk of 'community spirit' and 'a sense of community'. When it comes to the concept of 'community care', Jones et al. point out the multitude of possible interpretations:

> To the politician 'community care' is a useful piece of rhetoric, to the sociologist it is a stick to beat institutional care with, to the civil servant it is a cheap alternative to institutional care which can be passed to the local authority for action or inaction, to the visionary it is a dream of the new society in which people really do care, to social service departments it is a nightmare of heightened public expectations and inadequate resources to meet them. (1983: 102)

Bayley (1973) made the distinction between care *in* the community and care *by* the community. During the 1980s to the present time, there has been increasing emphasis on care *by* the community. Government now refers to the 'mixed economy of welfare', meaning that care of people deemed to be dependent must be the shared responsibility of statutory services, voluntary services, neighbours and family (*Caring for People*, 1989). Abbott and Sapsford (1987) found, however, that over half the families in their sample of parents with children with learning difficulties received either no help or very insignificant help.

Disability frequently results in extra expense in terms, for example, of diet, heating, transport, washing, special toys and alterations to the home. This can lead to additional stress, especially as disabled people and those who assist them are often excluded from the employment market. Graham (1984) believes that community care is a euphemism for an under-resourced system and that it represents care on the cheap. Potential funding is tied up in the institutions which cannot be sold because they are still partially occupied. Inadequate community resources frequently lead to 'the revolving-door syndrome' where people continually move between hospital and home.

Although discussion of 'community care' usually focuses on the closure of large institutions, in reality most disabled people have always lived within the community, being assisted by their families. This caring role usually falls to close female relatives who receive little or no assistance from formal or informal services (Parker, 1993), although the role which men play in caring is now being recognized (Arber and Gilbert, 1989). Beardshaw refers to services for younger disabled people as the 'Cinderella of Cinderella services' (1988: 7).

Women, in particular, often feel compelled to become carers, and tend to feel guilty if they reject the role. This is due to the widespread belief, not only that it is their duty, but that to care is a central, almost biological, aspect of the female character. Parker (1993) found that informal help was limited when a carer was present, and that statutory help was given to men more readily than women. She found no evidence, except in one case, of children being over involved in care.

Dalley (1988) believes that the liberation of one disadvantaged group, for example disabled people, can lead to the exploitation of another, for example women. Morris (1991) and Keith (1992), however, think that views such as these alienate disabled people by disregarding their experiences and viewing them as 'the problem'. There is little recognition that people are dependent on each other, physically and psychologically, or that those who need care are frequently carers themselves. Ryan and Thomas (1987) and Potts and Fido (1991) describe how the more able residents of mental handicap hospitals played a large role in caring for the less able residents, and Atkinson and Williams (1990), and Walmsley (1993) describe how people with learning difficulties often play a large role in caring for others in the community. This is frequently because they are 'trapped' in the family home with no socially sanctioned reasons, such as work commitments, not to care. Walmsley states, 'It is easy to over-simplify caring, to see a "carer" and a "dependent" in every caring relationship . . . this is not always the case. There may be giving and taking, exploitation and opportunity, on both sides of the caring relationship,' (1993: 135).

For these and other reasons disabled people have rejected the terms 'care' and 'carers' in favour of 'assistance', 'enablers' and 'personal assistants'. Disabled people are often under tremendous strain when forced to rely on a single helper, especially if that person would rather be somewhere else, they may also be at risk of emotional and physical abuse (Morris, 1993b).

'Community' is an emotive word which, like 'family', conjures up a nostalgic picture of warmth, friendship and neighbourliness. Politicians exploit this image when talking of 'care in the community', though in reality ill and disabled people discharged from institutions often end up in hotel rooms, inadequate hostels or on the streets. Hudson (1991) provides a detailed analysis of the failure of deinstitutionalization for people with learning difficulties. It should be appreciated that the situation of disabled people in 'normal' society is frequently highly abnormal due to prejudice, adverse stereotyping, and the difficulty of adapting to an environment designed for non-disabled living. For life in 'the community' to be successful, therefore, the wider social and economic environment, in terms of housing, employment, transport, education and leisure facilities, must change to accommodate disabled people. Hicks states:

> A bridge needs to be built between the invisible world of family care and the public one of long-stay, institutional care. A middle way needs to be found which neither confines each carer to her private hell nor condemns our elderly and disabled population to being looked after exclusively by the state and its institutions. (1988: 252)

Housing

There is a serious shortage of wheelchair-accessible housing in Great Britain, and considerable homelessness among disabled people. Morris (1990), in her survey of 21 local authorities in England and Wales, found that homelessness among physically disabled people rose by 92 per cent between 1980 and 1986 compared with 57 per cent among non-disabled people. There was little recognition within local authorities that disabled people become homeless, and little consultation with them. Only three housing departments had a written policy on the needs of disabled people, and only two were in regular contact with social service departments. Home owners were often excluded from receiving any assistance, leaving them in totally unsuitable accommodation. Morris states:

> Residential care is still considered as inevitable for many disabled people. Sometimes this is a solution of last resort, because of the lack of housing and support services. Most often there is little awareness of either the potential for independent living or how its denial is a denial of a basic human right. (1993b: 141)

Hurst (1992) believes that all housing should be built with certain items such as wide doorways and a downstairs toilet. She points out that features such as these are ones which most people, disabled or not, would welcome; many of these features have been introduced by law in Sweden (Ratzka, 1992). Dunn (1990) demonstrates that accessible housing provides disabled people with greater safety, privacy and independence, allowing them to participate more fully in community life and paid employment. It also has a beneficial effect on other members of the family. (For further details of housing and disabled people, the reader is referred to Laurie, 1991.)

Independent living

For disabled people who require help in everyday living, solutions other than institutions or assistance by relatives do exist and ought to be expanded. These include fostering and 'boarding out' schemes and the Crossroads Care Attendant Scheme, which provides trained personnel to assist disabled people in their own homes. Day hospitals and day centres have also gone some way towards providing assistance, and schemes where ordinary families live independently of, but in close proximity to, disabled people and assist them in exchange for a wage, operate in some parts of the country (Davis, 1981). Community Service Volunteers provide young people to assist disabled people on a twenty-four hour basis. Sheltered accommodation, where a warden is on call, is another example.

Although solutions such as these can be a considerable improvement on both institutional living and assistance by relatives, they still leave disabled people fitting in with other people's schedules with little control of their own lives. Straughair and Fawcitt (1992) found, for example, that most of the young people with arthritis they interviewed felt it was not possible for them to leave the parental home because there was no substitute for the support and flexibility their parents provided. Others felt they could not move because of the financial benefits their parents would lose and the money they had expended on adaptations.

Many disabled people have found that the only way of achieving a satisfactory lifestyle is to hire and train their own assistants. The Independent Living Fund, set up in 1988, provided disabled people with this opportunity, but the applications made drastically exceeded government expectations and the fund was closed to new applicants in 1992. Some disabled people use their own income, along with disability benefits, to buy their own assistance, but this option is out of the question for people whose income is low (Barnes, 1991).

Morris (1993b) interviewed fifty disabled people, between the ages of 19 and 55, who were living in the community. Some were relying on statutory services while others received direct payment to hire their own assistants. Those who relied on statutory services found that these were unresponsive to their needs and created major restrictions in their lives, dictating, for example, the time they went to bed and how frequently they bathed. Professional workers created barriers too by the specificity of their roles. Disabled people were sometimes compelled to emphasize or even exaggerate their impairments in order to get the help they required; one disabled person, for example, was forced to emphasize his incontinence in order to get help with washing his clothes. This is an example of fitting the client to the service. Morris states, 'A failure of statutory bodies to provide services which enable disabled people to carry on their daily lives and engage in ordinary personal relationships creates a very poor quality of life and undermines human and civil rights' (1993b: 26).

Finding information about the options available was also a major difficulty. Disability organizations and other disabled people were the most common sources of advice on moving out of institutions and employing personal assistants. D'Aboville (1991) believes that disabled people who have set up their own personal assistance schemes have done so in spite, rather than because, of the involvement of professionals.

The interviewees in Morris's study who received direct payments for hiring and training their own assistants had an entirely different experience. It enabled them to participate in society as they wished, and for some it permitted them to engage in paid employment, to support their parents, and to bring up their own children. Receiving some paid help from outside the family was seen by most disabled people as crucial to maintaining equality of relationships within the family. Morris states:

> Those people who had the money to pay for personal assistance were generally able to have the control over their lives which was not possible for those solely reliant on other services or on family and friends. This kind of control was important not only for those who lived on their own, but also for those people living with partners, parents and/or children. (1993b: 37)

Some of the disabled people interviewed stressed that they did not want assistants with professional qualifications because they wanted to train them in their own way. One person said, 'we feel that the less experience they have the better . . . we know what needs doing, *they* don't need to know, they just need to be told' (1993b: 33).

The only way of enabling disabled people to have the choices which non-disabled people take for granted is to introduce a fully comprehensive direct payment system, but as Morris (1993b) points out this has no place in the community care reforms which advocate resource-led assessments of disabled people by professionals, and the purchase of 'care' by managers. Morris states:

> The ideology of caring which is at the heart of current community care policies can only result in institutionalisation within the community, unless politicians and professionals understand and identify with the philosophy and aims of the independent living movement. Independent living is a human and civil rights issue; community care confines people to the four walls of their own home, preventing them from fully participating in personal relationships and society, condoning the emotional and physical abuse which goes on behind closed doors. (1993: 43)

(For personal accounts of disabled people hiring and managing their own assistants, the reader is referred to Briggs (1993) and Macfarlane (1993).)

Oliver and Zarb (1992) carried out some similar research among sixteen disabled people in Greenwich who were receiving direct payment for personal assistance. Employing their own workers improved the quality of their lives enormously enabling them to work and to expand their social and leisure activities. Thirteen people had found out about the scheme through the Greenwich Association of Disabled People and only one through a social worker. The Greenwich Association of Disabled People also helped half of the disabled people to recruit their assistants. Considerable help may be required to manage personal assistants on an interpersonal as well as a practical level, for as Rae points out disabled people 'are conditioned not to structure other people's lives' (1989: 10).

Oliver and Zarb demonstrate by detailed analysis that money can be saved by providing disabled people with direct payments, and that the necessary resources can easily be found by switching them from other areas. They state:

> The success of Personal Assistance Schemes in allowing users to control how their support needs are met, provides a good model for the empowerment of disabled people by demonstrating that—given genuine choice and adequate resources—disabled people are able to exercise control over their lives and reduce for themselves their enforced dependency on inadequate services. (1992: 13).

Morris (1993) is also of the opinion that current working practices tie up money in ways which are incompatible with independent living. (For further information on community care, the reader is referred to Bornat et al. 1993).

Conclusion

The Manchester Coalition of Disabled People states that 'everyone has a right to choose how and where they want to live, and who they live with' and that 'Nobody should have to choose between being a burden to their family or living in a residential institution'. They believe that 'those who support and look after disabled people have rights and needs' and that 'disabled people and people who provide them with care do not have to suffer at each other's expense' (undated: 1). The assistance provided for disabled people in Great Britain today is inadequate, restrictive, patchy and largely unimaginative. Morris concludes that 'Current community care policies can only result in institutionalisation in the community unless politicians and professionals understand and identify with the philosophy and aims of the independent living movement' (1993: 179).

Therapists and nurses work with disabled people in a variety of institutional and community settings. It is important that they are aware of the full range of options possible and the advantages and disadvantages of each for any particular person. They must think and act broadly and flexibly, outside the medical model, to avoid inadvertently restricting and alienating the very people they are trying to assist. Most of all they must consult disabled people and their organizations.

A suitable place to live is of the utmost importance to the happiness and well-being of disabled people. Yet in reality, despite many innovative schemes and considerable improvement, the choice is still too often between the family and an institution. This is unacceptable and a situation which therapists and nurses can play their part in changing.

References

Abbott, P. and Sapsford, R. (1987) *Community Care for Mentally Handicapped Children*, Open University Press, Milton Keynes

Abercrombie, N., Hill, S. and Turner, B. (1988) *Dictionary of Sociology*, Penguin Books, Harmondsworth

Arber, S. and Gilbert, N. (1989) Men: the forgotten carers. *Sociology*, **23** (1), 111–118

Atkinson, D. and Williams, F. (1990) *Know Me As I am: An Anthology of Prose, Poetry and Art by People with Learning Difficulties*, Hodder & Stoughton, Sevenoaks

Barnes, C. (1991) *Disabled People in Britain and Discrimination*, Hurst & Company, London

Bayley, M. J. (1973) *Mental Handicap and Community Care*, Routledge & Kegan Paul, London

Beardshaw, V. (1988) *Last on the List: Community Services for People with Physical Disabilities*, King's Fund Institute, London

Booth, T. and Statham, J. (1982) *The Nature of Special Education*, Croom Helm, London

Bornat, J., Pereira, C., Pilgrim, D. and Williams, F. (eds) (1993) *Community Care*, Macmillan, London

Briggs, L. (1993) Striving for independence. In *Disabling Barriers—Enabling Environments*, (eds J. Swain, V. Finkelstein, S. French and M. Oliver), Sage, London

Caring for People: Community Care in the Next Decade and Beyond (1989) HMSO, London

The Coalition and Care in the Community (undated) Manchester Coalition of Disabled People, Manchester

Committee of Enquiry into the Education of Handicapped Children and Young People (1978) *Special Educational Needs*, Warnock Report, HMSO, London

Cooke, M. (1987) Part of the institution. *Nursing Times*, **83 (23)**, 25–27

d'Aboville, E. (1991) Social work in an organisation of disabled people. In *Social Work, Disabled People and Disabling Environments*, (ed. M. Oliver), Jessica Kingsley, London

Dalley, G. (1988) *Ideologies of Caring*, Macmillan, London

Davidson, N. (1987) Community care or community neglect? In *A Question of Care*, (ed. N. Davidson), Michael Joseph, London

Davis, K. (1981) 28–38 Grove Road: accommodation and care in a community setting. In *Handicap in a Social World*, (eds A. Brechin, P. Liddiard and J. Swain), Hodder & Stoughton, Sevenoaks

Davis, K. (1993) The crafting of good clients. In *Disabling Barriers—Enabling Environments*, (eds J. Swain, V. Finkelstein, S. French and M. Oliver), Sage, London

Dunn, P. A. (1990) The impact of the housing environment upon the ability of disabled people to live independently. *Disability, Handicap and Society*, **5 (1)**, 37–52

Finkelstein, V. (1991) Disability: an administrative challenge. In *Social Work, Disabled People and Disabling Environments*, Jessica Kingsley, London

Ford, S. (1987) Into the outside. *Nursing Times*, **83 (20)**, 40–42

French S. (1992) Memories of school 1958–1962. In *Living Proof*, (ed. S. O'Keefe), The Royal National Institute for the Blind, London

Goffman, I. (1961) *Asylums*, Penguin Books, Harmondsworth

Graham, H. (1984) *Women, Health and the Family*, Macmillan, London

Harrison, J. (1987) *Severe Physical Disability*, Cassell, London

Harrison, J. (1993) Medical responsibilities to disabled people. In *Disabling Barriers—Enabling Environments*, (eds J. Swain, V. Finkelstein, S. French and M. Oliver), Sage, London

Hicks, C. (1988) *Who Cares?* Virago Press, London

Holmes, B. and Johnson, A. (1988) *Cold Comfort*, Souvenir Press London

Hudson, B. (1991) Deinstitutionalization: what went wrong? *Disability, Handicap and Society*, **6 (1)**, 21–36

Humphries, S. and Gordon, P. (1992) *Out of Sight: The Experience of Disability 1900–1950*, Northcote House, Plymouth

Hunt, J. (1992) The disabled people's movement between 1960–1986 and its effect upon the development of community support services. M Sc Dissertation by independent study. University of East London

Hurst, R. (1992) Independent living, civil rights and housing. In *Building Our Lives: Housing, Independent Living and Disabled People*, (ed. L. Laurie), Shelter, London

Illich, I. (1976) *Limits to Medicine*, Penguin, Harmondsworth

Jones, K., Brown, J. and Bradshaw, J. (1983) *Issues in Social Policy*, Routledge & Kegan Paul, London

Keith, L. (1992) Who cares wins? Women, caring, and disability. *Disability, Handicap and Society* **7 (2)**, 167–176

Ladd, P. (1990) Language oppression and hearing impairment. In the book of readings of the disability equality training pack *Disability—Changing Practice* (K665x), Open University, Milton Keynes

Laing, R. D. (1967) *The Politics of Experience and the Bird of Paradise*, Penguin Books, Harmondsworth

Laurie, L. (1991) (ed.) *Building Our Lives: Housing, Independent Living and Disabled People*, Shelter, London

McConkey, R. (1987) *Who Cares? Community Involvement with Handicapped People*, Souvenir Press, London

Macfarlane, A. (1993) The right to make choices. In *Community Care*, (1993) (eds P. J. Bornat, C. Pereira, D. Pilgrim and F. Williams), Macmillan, London

McLeod, W. T. (1986) (ed.) *The Collins Paperback English Dictionary*, Collins, London

Madge, N. and Fassam, M. (1982) *Ask the Children*, Batsford, London

Marchant, R. and Page, M. (1992) *Bridging the Gap*, National Society for the Prevention of Cruelty to Children, London

Meadow, W. P. (1980) *Deafness and Child Development*, Arnold, London

Mittler, P. (1979) *People Not Patients: Problems and Policies in Mental Handicap*, Methuen, London

Morris, J. (1990) *Our Homes Our Right: Housing, Independent Living, and Physically Disabled People*, Shelter, London

Morris, J. (1991) *Pride Against Prejudice*, The Women's Press, London

Morris, J. (1993) *Community Care or Independent Living?* Joseph Rowntree Foundation, London

Oliver, M. and Zarb, G. (1992) *Personal Assistance Schemes*, Greenwich Association of Disabled People, London

Orford, J. (1980) Institutional Climates, In *Psychology and Medicine*, (ed. D. Griffiths), Macmillan, London

Oswin, M. (1978) *Holes in the Welfare Net*, Bedford Square Press, London

Parker, G. (1993) *With this Body: Caring and Disability in Marriage*, Open University Press, Buckingham

Potts, M. and Fido, R. (1991) *'A Fit Person to be Removed': Personal Accounts of Life in a Mental Deficiency Institution*, Northcote House, Plymouth

Rae, A. (1989) Enablers not carers. *Disability Now*, October

Ratzka, A. (1992) The Swedish experience. In *Building Our Lives: Housing, Independent Living and Disabled People*, (ed. L. Laurie), Shelter, London

Richman, J. (1987) *Medicine and Health*, Longman, London

Ryan, J. and Thomas, F. (1987) *The Politics of Mental Handicap*, Free Association Books, London

Scott, R. A., (1969) *The Making of Blind Men*, Russell Sage Foundation, New York

Sedgwick, J. (1989) Dressed with dignity. *Nursing Times*, **85 (48)**, 30–31

Shearer, A. (1982) *Living Independently*, Centre for the Environment of the Handicapped and The King's Fund Centre, London

Straughair, S. and Fawcitt, S. (1992) *The Road Towards Independence: The Experiences of Young People with Arthritis in the 1990s*, Arthritis Care, London

Szasz, T. S. (1961) *The Myth of Mental Illness*, Harper & Row, New York

Townsend, P. (1962) *The Last Refuge*, Routledge & Kegan Paul, London

Tully, K. (1986) *Improving Residential Life for Disabled People*, Churchill Livingstone, London

Vaizey, J. (1959) Scenes from Institutional Life, cited in *Issues in Social Policy*, (1983) (eds K. Jones, J. Brown and J. Bradshaw), Routledge & Kegan Paul, London

Wade, B. and Moore, M. (1993) *Experiencing Special Education*, Open University Press, Buckingham

Walmsley, J. (1993) Contradictions in caring: reciprocity and interdependence. *Disability, Handicap and Society*, **8 (2)**, 129–141

Westcott, H. L. (1991) *Institutional Abuse of Children—From Research to Policy: A Review*, National Society for the Prevention of Cruelty to Children, London

Westcott, H. L. (1993) *Abuse of Children and Adults with Disabilities*, National Society for the Prevention of Cruelty to Children, London

Wilkinson, D. (1987) Busy doing nothing. *Nursing Times*, **83 (23)**, 30–31

10

Researching disability

Sally French

It has been seen in previous chapters that disability is generally defined in an individualistic, medicalized fashion, as a property of people with impairments; most research on disability reflects this individualistic orientation. In contrast to this, many disabled people and their organizations view disability in terms of physical, social and attitudinal barriers which could be removed if the personal and political will to do so was present, and believe that research should reflect this orientation.

Defining disability in research

The way disability is defined will set the tone of any research project. The researcher may take an individualistic, medicalized stance, suggesting that the impairment, and the impairment alone, creates the disability. It is possible, however, to take a social view of disability where it is defined in terms of the barriers disabled people face – the library steps blocking the wheelchair user's entry, the cluttered pavements impeding the progress of those with visual impairments, and the numerous social and physical obstacles barring disabled people's access to employment, education and housing.

If an individualistic stance to disability is taken, the questions posed by the researcher will be based on impairment rather than the measures which could be taken by society to alleviate or eliminate disability. It obviously makes an enormous difference whether the questions are posed in terms of 'what people cannot do' rather than in terms of how society can be changed to enable disabled people to participate fully within it. Oliver (1990) highlights this point by substituting the individualistic questions used in the government's OPCS surveys of disability with questions reflecting a social orientation. For example, in place of the question 'What complaint causes your difficulty in holding, gripping and turning things?', he writes 'What defects in the design of everyday equipment like jars, bottles and tins, causes your difficulty in holding, gripping and turning them?', and in place of the question 'Did you move here because of your health problem/disability?', he writes 'What inadequacies in your housing caused you to move here?' (Oliver, 1990). Oliver asks:

> might it not be a better aim for researchers to construct indicators of disabling environments rather than continue to count the number of disabled people? Indeed, how much more interesting would it be to construct a disability index for each local authority, for example, so that Brent could be compared with Camden or Kent to see which local authority had the most and which had the least disabling policies. (1993: 66)

In the OPCS surveys (Martin et al., 1988; Bone and Meltzer, 1989), the severity of an individual's disability is conceptualized as the extent to which his or her performance of everyday activities is limited by impairment; ten severity levels are presented from which the judges can choose. Their decisions are, however, made with no regard to social context or individual circumstances. It is stated, for example, that 'not being able to walk is clearly more limiting that being able to walk only 50 yards' (Martin et al. 1988: 50). However, the reverse may be the case if the criteria for the provision of a wheelchair is the *lack* of ability to walk this distance; a disabled person using a wheelchair may have far *less* difficulty covering this stretch than someone walking independently or using crutches. Abberley (1991) is of the opinion that any attempt to discriminate finely different levels of severity is nothing more than the subjective opinions of mainly non-disabled 'experts'.

The OPCS surveys are based upon the definitions of disability provided by the *International Classification of Impairments Disabilities and Handicaps* (ICIDH) which were first published by the World Health Organization in 1980. This system was used despite the fact that the British Council of Organizations of Disabled People had rejected it because of its insistence that disability arises from impairment (see chapter 1).

Further problems arise in the OPCS surveys when the severity of one impairment is compared with that of another. Is it really more disabling not to be able to touch ones knees and then straighten than to fail to recognize a friend across a room, or twice as severe as the inability to hear a quiet voice across a room, as the OPCS survey suggests? (Martin et al., 1988). As disabled people so frequently point out, disability has more to do with the organization of society, including the status and income of disabled people themselves, than their impairments. The OPCS surveys do acknowledge this in part by stating that 'some people with impairments may, as a result of aids and appliances, have only a very minor level of disability and, as such, fall below the threshold level' (Martin et al., 1988). Examples are given of spectacles, pacemakers and medication eliminating disability, but these ideas are not applied to more severe impairments.

Many questions in the OPCS surveys are structured in such a way that presenting them to people with long-standing impairments, and requiring an answer, sets them an impossible task. Abberley suggests that 'to ask someone if they have difficulty is to ask them to make a social comparison which a disabled person is in a particularly unsuitable position to do' (1991: 164). If people who have been visually impaired from birth, for example, are asked how difficult they find it to read newsprint, how can they answer accurately without knowledge of how difficult those around them find the activity? A meaningful answer would also be far more complex than a closed 'yes/no' response could accommodate, for their ability may have everything to do with which newspaper they are attempting to read, the size and boldness of the print, the lighting conditions and whether or not their visual aids are to hand. Because many disabled people have never experienced 'normality' they have a great tendency to under-report the difficulties they experience (Patrick, 1989; Anderson et al., 1989). Abberley (1991) points out that disabled people have no 'normal' baseline to measure their efforts against.

Researchers can choose, therefore, to pose questions suggesting that the disability is contained within the disabled individual or, in contrast, those which suggest that disability is a social phenomenon. Abberley states that 'it is a political decision, conscious or otherwise, to employ questions of the first type rather than the second' (1991: 158). If a social view of disability is taken, then it becomes a political issue, a matter of civil rights and not of medical needs. Abberley expands his case further, stating that, 'Attempts to depoliticise the unavoidably political, to examine the complex and subtle through crude and simplistic measures indicates by negative example some of the things that good research in this area, and indeed any research, requires' (1991: 174). Even basic 'facts', such as the number of disabled people residing in a given place, are based upon the criteria used to define disability which, in turn, may reflect the interests of the researchers or their funders.

It is unfortunate that, despite such serious flaws, the results of large and prestigious disability surveys, like those conducted and sponsored by government, are frequently used to inform and shape social policy and professional practice. It should be remembered, however, that professional practice frequently has no sound research or theoretical base. Although this situation is sometimes justifiable, professional practice based on little or no research or theoretical underpinnings can do serious harm. Examples include the practice of preventing deaf children from using sign language, which causes them social and emotional harm (Volterra, 1991), and the practice of preventing visually-impaired children from using their sight, which was the custom in special schools until the Second World War (Corley et al., 1989). Finkelstein states:

> None of the existing service approaches to disability were set up on the basis of an in-depth understanding of what disability is about. . . . The body of knowledge which has been created by service provision which enables professionals in the field of disability to call themselves experts came into being without any real attempt to understand this subject. (1990a: 3)

Another example of professional practice with flimsy theoretical underpinnings is 'conductive education' (the Peto technique). Despite the expansion and professionalization of this treatment approach for people with neurological conditions, sound research and a firm theoretical base are practically nil (Oliver, 1989; Rowat, 1993). Kinsman states that, 'The theoretical background is not well known, for Peto wrote little about conductive education, and there have been few publications from the institute and these mention little about the underlying theory' (1989: 420). Recent findings on the effectiveness of conductive education from Birmingham University have proved disappointing (Barstow et al., 1993a, 1993b). The method focuses entirely on impairment and striving for 'normality', a stance which has been strongly criticized by many disabled people and their organizations (Oliver, 1990; Finkelstein, 1990b and 1993; French, 1993).

Research as oppression

> Disabled people have come to see research as a violation of their experience, as irrelevant to their needs and as failing to improve their material circumstances and quality of life. (Oliver 1992: 105)

Oliver contends that research is an activity undertaken by those who have power upon those who do not; it is certainly the case that far less research is directed at those with the means to safeguard their privacy (Oliver, 1992). Disabled people and their organizations tend to interpret disability in terms of political oppression rather than random personal tragedy (Barton, 1988). Thus if researchers choose to reflect an individualistic stance to disability they and their research may serve to oppress disabled people by depoliticizing the political. Abberley states that 'Information gathered on the basis of an oppressive theory, unless handled with circumspection, is itself one of the mechanisms of oppression' (1992: 154). If isolated disabled people are asked questions about their disabilities posed in terms of impairment by someone in authority, this will only serve to disempower them by reinforcing the notion that the problems they experience are 'their' problems. It can be seen that research is not a value-neutral activity. Oliver (1983) makes the point that few, if any, studies have started out with the assumption that disability is not a problem.

Keith draws our attention to the lessons we can learn from feminist research with regard to the underlying and often erroneous assumptions on which research is frequently based. She states 'Feminist research has taught us about the ways in which our own experiences, and our everyday lived reality, colour and shape our interpretations of the social world. It also shapes what gets researched and written about' (1992: 170). Keith (1992) points out, with regard to research on carers, that only one version of a set of events has been studied (that of the carers) which has served to alienate disabled and older people by disregarding their experiences and viewing them as 'the problem'. There is very little recognition that we are all, to some degree, dependent on others, and that those who need 'care' are often carers themselves (Morris, 1991; Morris, 1993a; Parker, 1993; Walmsley, 1993). Morris believes that researchers 'have few tools with which to understand our subjective reality because our own definitions of the experience of disability are missing from the general culture' (1992: 165). She believes that researchers need to develop an understanding of the subjective reality of disabled people and to turn the focus of their research towards the oppressors (Morris, 1993b).

Disabled people are sometimes denied any opportunity to take part in research, even as 'subjects', because researchers are not willing or able to make their research accessible. Baker-Shenk and Kyle (1990) give a detailed account of the conflicts which arise when hearing researchers attempt to study deaf people and their language. Ways must be found of encouraging and enabling disabled people to carry out research into their own situation, and for research practice to be shaped to ensure their full participation. Jones and Pullen (1992), a hearing and a deaf researcher, have demonstrated the value of using interviewing techniques suited to deaf people. They point out the importance of understanding the differing meanings of time, touch, visual information and language within deaf and hearing cultures.

Disabled people are the most impoverished section of the community and may feel that money is wasted on research when they could have provided the information themselves directly (Zarb, 1992). Zarb urges researchers to be honest about the professional, academic and financial benefits which may accrue to them when they undertake research into disability. It is important that whatever research is done will benefit disabled people in ways which they perceive as useful. As Oliver states:

> the major issue on the research agenda for the 1990s should be; do researchers wish to join with disabled people to use their expertise and

skills in their struggle against oppression or do they wish to continue
to use these skills and expertise in ways in which disabled people find
oppressive? (1992: 102)

What sort of disability research is needed?

It can be seen from the above account that a major problem regarding
disability research is that, other than being 'subjects', disabled people
are rarely involved in it, and that this situation leads to inappropriate
questions being asked and unsuitable services being developed.
There has been an underlying assumption that disability is the result
of impairment, and that disabled people are dependent and in need
of cure or care. Many disabled people and their organizations now
believe that a more participatory style of research should be adopted
where disabled people are consulted at every stage of the research
process, and assisted and encouraged to carry out research into
disability issues themselves.

Participatory and emancipatory research

Participatory research is an approach which has been evolving in
recent years, particularly in the developing countries. Chambers refers to it as 'a new paradigm', 'a coherent and mutually supportive
pattern of concepts, values, methods and actions amenable to wide
application' (1986: 1). Participatory research aims to involve, at every
stage of the research process—choice of topics, methods, evaluation
and dissemination—those towards whom research is directed, people
who Chambers describes as 'the last'. These may include disabled
people, patients and rural village dwellers in developing countries.
   There is no place for 'subjects' or passive co-operation in this
approach, instead everyone involved is an *active* participant. The
expertise and talents of everyone are utilized to the full, with training
being given if necessary; the approach does not, however, reject
expert knowledge or help from outside, rather it aims to make traditional research more effective and meaningful.
   Any research method can be used in participatory research, but the
emphasis is on those which are eclectic, inventive and flexible, giving
room for new ideas to emerge and allowing for changes of plan and
direction as the research proceeds. Methods are adapted to suit the
particular situation and the people involved, rather than forcing ideas
into a fixed method. With traditional research, complex issues are
sometimes simplified or avoided because the methods are too rigid
to accommodate them.

A major aim of participatory research is to provide educational opportunities to those who are so often at the receiving end of research directed by 'experts'. This, it is hoped, will have the effect of increasing their skills, self-reliance and self-confidence, leading to social action which they perceive to be relevant and important. It is a democratic means of accelerating social change and reducing exploitation.

The widespread effects that Chambers (1986) believes participatory research may have are summarized below:

1. It breaks down the mystique surrounding research.
2. It balances grassroots and macro-analysis.
3. It ensures that the problems researched are perceived as problems by the people to whom the research is directed.
4. It makes use of personal experience and 'lay' knowledge.
5. It helps to develop self-confidence, self-reliance and skills in people to whom the research is directed.
6. It spans the cultures of academia and practice, thereby addressing both academic and practical issues.
7. It encourages democratic interaction and transfer of power, thus reducing exploitation.
8. It challenges the way knowledge is produced.
9. It gives a sense of collective responsibility.
10. It enables people to view their situation in a wider context.
11. It avoids the fragmentation of knowledge, providing a holistic approach.
12. It enables people to analyse their situation and take action.

Participatory research aims not only to investigate important issues, but to facilitate fundamental social change. People at the bottom of any hierarchy rarely have sufficient power to generate knowledge, indeed such power is usually held by those furthest from the situation. As Brechin states, 'Research tends to be owned and controlled by researchers, or by those who, in turn, own and control the researchers' (1993: 73). The result of all this is that the issues investigated may have little relevance to those who are being researched, thereby erecting social barriers and hindering meaningful social change.

Some of the problems Chambers (1986) considers are associated with more traditional research approaches are summarized below:

1. Relevant modes of analysis are neglected. Methods tend to be rigidly adhered to and may determine both problem and solution.
2. The problems investigated may be of interest only to the researchers and other 'outsiders', and may be inappropriate to 'real' situations.

3. Traditional research tends to undervalue the people to whom it is directed by not enlisting their active involvement.
4. Action tends to follow published work, which is often out of date. Any action which follows usually depends on the judgement of 'experts'.
5. Traditional research tends to be costly.
6. The research is influenced by forces which favour the strong and powerful.
7. Certain issues are neglected because they are not the priority of any profession, thus gaps are left in the knowledge.

A shift of emphasis of the magnitude required to change traditional research to participatory research would obviously require enormous attitudinal and behavioural change on the part of researchers. It is important that researchers understand the meaning of participatory research and do not involve disabled people in a superficial or token-istic way. As Oliver points out, 'researchers have benefited by taking the experience (of disabled people), rendering a faithful account of it and then moving on to better things while the disabled subjects remain in exactly the same social situation they did before the research began' (Oliver 1992: 109).

Zarb (1992) draws a distinction between 'participatory research' and 'emancipatory research' believing that research cannot be emancipatory unless it is empowering, but that empowerment cannot be *given* but rather must be *taken*. Talking of research into disability he states:

> Participatory research which involves disabled people in a meaningful way is perhaps a pre-requisite to emancipatory research in the sense that researchers can learn from disabled people and vice versa, and that it paves the way for researchers to make themselves 'available' to disabled people—but it is no more than that. Simply increasing partici-pation and involvement will never by itself constitute emancipatory research unless and until it is disabled people themselves who are controlling the research and deciding who should be involved and how. (1992: 128)

Morris agrees, believing that emancipatory research 'must be part of disabled people's struggle to take over ownership of the definition of oppression' (1991: 162).

Zarb (1992) believes that research can, by asking questions such as the following, be categorized with regard to how far it is 'participatory' or 'emancipatory':

Participatory research
1. Who controls what the research is about and how it is done?
2. How far are disabled people involved in the research process?

3. Can disabled people influence future directions?
4. Are there pathways by which disabled people can be critical of the research?

Emancipatory research
1. How alienating is the research practice for researchers and disabled people participating in it?
2. What opportunities does the research create for self-reflection and mutual sharing of experience and understanding between researchers and disabled people?
3. What happens to the products of the research?
4. Does the research have the potential to empower disabled people?

Zarb points out that researchers rarely have total control of the research process because they have to satisfy the funders. He states:

> it is usually impossible to make an absolutely explicit statement to the effect that the participants' interests will be the only ones the research will address. The reality is that we have to pay attention to the interests and priorities of funders. (Zarb 1992: 129)

Much can be done to involve disabled people in research, however, and guidelines have been devised to help researchers involved in disability research decide which bodies to approach for funding. (Guidelines for funding applications to undertake disability research, 1992.)

Conclusion

Participatory and emancipatory research may seem somewhat removed from the everyday world of the practising therapist or nurse, but these practitioners are in a unique position to involve disabled people in research which affects their lives. Morris believes that non-disabled researchers should be the allies of disabled people, that they should ask 'where are the disabled researchers? students? academics?' (1992: 164), and that they should challenge discrimination and ensure that the research they conduct empowers disabled people. As Oliver states:

> The late twentieth century has seen a crisis of these productions of disability because disabled people have penetrated the medical and individual ideologies underpinning them. What's more, having done so, they are now engaged in a struggle to produce disability as social oppression. As this struggle continues and disabled people grow in strength, the crisis in disability production will deepen and researchers

will be forced to ask the question Howard Becker asked thirty years ago: Whose side are you on? (1992: 101).

The way in which disability has been researched has become a major issue for disabled people and their organizations in recent years. In 1991 a series of seminars, sponsored by the Joseph Rowntree Foundation, took place, where disabled and non-disabled researchers had the opportunity to debate this issue in considerable depth; this culminated in a conference 'Researching Disability: Setting the Agenda for Change' which took place in 1992.

Disabled people are being empowered by the disability movement; the question is, can research become part of that empowerment?

References

Abberley, P. (1991) The Significance of the OPCS disability surveys. In *Social Work, Disabled People and Disabling Environments*, (ed. M. Oliver), Jessica Kingsley, London

Abberley, P. (1992) Counting us out: a discussion of the OPCS disability surveys. *Disability, Handicap and Society*, **7 (2)**, 139–156

Anderson, J., Bush, J. and Berry, C. (1989) Performance versus capacity: a conflict for classifying function for health status measurements. Cited in *Disablement in the Community*, (eds D. L. Patrick and H. Peach), Oxford University Press, Oxford

Baker-Shenk, C. and Kyle, J. G. (1990) Research with deaf people: issues and conflicts. *Disability, Handicap and Society*, **5 (1)**, 65–75

Barstow, P., Cochrane, R. and Hur, J. (1993a) *Evaluation of Conductive Education (Part 1)*, HMSO, London

Barstow, P., Cochrane, R. and Hur, J. (1993b) *Evaluation of Conductive Education (Part 2)*, HMSO, London

Barton, L. (1988) Research and practice: the need for alternative perspectives. In *The Politics of Special Educational Needs*, (ed. L. Barton), The Falmer Press, London

Bone, M. and Meltzer, H. (1989) *The Prevalence of Disability Among Children*, OPCS Surveys of Disability in Great Britain, Report 3, Office of Population Censuses and Surveys, London

Brechin, A. (1993) 'Sharing'. In *Reflecting on Research Practice: Issues in Health and Social Welfare*, (eds P. Shakespeare, D. Atkinson and S. French), Open University Press, Buckingham

Chambers, R. (1986) *Normal Professionalism: New Paradigms and Development*, Discussion Paper 227, Institute of Development Studies, Brighton

Corley, G., Robinson, D. and Lockett, S. (1989) *Partially Sighted Children*, NFER/Nelson, London

Finkelstein, V. (1990a) Services for clients or clients for services? Paper given at the annual conference of the North Regional Association of the Blind, 18 October

Finkelstein, V. (1990b) A tale of two cities. *Therapy Weekly*, **16 (34)**, 6–7

Finkelstein, V. (1993) Being disabled, Workbook 2 of the Open University course *The Disabling Society* (K665), The Open University, Milton Keynes

French, S. (1993) Dismantling the barriers. Workbook 3 of the Open University course *The Disabling Society* (K665), The Open University, Milton Keynes

Guidelines for funding applications to undertake disability research. (1992) *Disability, Handicap and Society*, **7 (3)**, 279–280

International Classification of Impairments, Disabilities and Handicaps (1980), The World Health Organization

Jones, L. and Pullen, G. (1992) Cultural differences: deaf and hearing researchers working together. *Disability, Handicap and Society*, **7 (2)**, 189–196

Keith, L. (1992) Who cares wins? Women, caring and disability. *Disability, Handicap and Society*, **7 (2)**, 167–176

Kinsman, R. (1989) A conductive education approach to stroke patients at Barnet General Hospital. *Physiotherapy*, **75**, 418–420

Martin, J., Meltzer, H. and Eliot, D. (1988) *The Prevalence of Disability Among Adults*, OPCS Survey of Disability, Report 1, Office of Population Censuses and Surveys, London

Morris, J. (1991) *Pride Against Prejudice*, The Women's Press, London

Morris, J. (1992) Personal and political: a feminist perspective on researching physical disability. *Disability, Handicap and Society*, **7 (2)**, 157–166

Morris, J. (1993a) *Independent Lives? Community Care and Disabled People*, Macmillan, London

Morris, J. (1993b) Feminism and disability. *Feminist Review*, Spring, **43**, 57–70

Oliver, M. (1983) *Social Work and Disabled People*, Macmillan, London

Oliver, M. (1989) Conductive education: if it wasn't so sad it would be funny. *Disability, Handicap and Society*, **4**, 197–200

Oliver, M. (1990) *The Politics of Disablement*, Macmillan, London

Oliver, M. (1992) Changing the social relations of research production. *Disability, Handicap and Society*, **7 (2)**, 101–114

Oliver, M. (1993) Re-defining disability: a challenge to research. In *Disabling Barriers—Enabling Environments*, (eds. J. Swain, V. Finkelstein, S. French and M. Oliver), Sage, London

Parker, G. (1993) *With this Body: Caring and Disability in Marriage*, Open University Press, Buckingham

Patrick, D. L. (1989) Screening for disability. In *Disablement in the*

Community, (eds. D. L. Patrick and H. Peach), Oxford University Press, Oxford

Researching disability: setting the agenda for change. (1992) National Disability Conference, Kensington and Chelsea Town Hall, 1 June 1992, London

Rowat, A. (1993) Conductive education: does it work? *Disability Now*, June, 13

Walmsley, J. (1993) Contradictions in caring: reciprocity and interdependence. *Disability Handicap and Society*, **8 (2)**, 129–141

Volterra, V. (1991) What sign language research can teach us about language acquisition. In *Constructing Deafness*, (eds S. Gregory and G. M. Hartley), Pinter Publishers, London

Zarb, G. (1992) On the road to Damascus: first steps towards changing the relations of disability research production. *Disability, Handicap and Society*, **7 (2)**, 125–138

11

Learning disability: overcoming the barriers?

Jan Walmsley

Introduction

> There's plenty things we could do but we don't get the chance. The only one thing that's stopping us really is we're working in here and we're labelled and that's what 'cos I hate being in here. If you're in here you get labelled as handicapped. (Atkinson and Williams, 1990: 152)

The speaker, a student at an adult training centre in Scotland, attributes the problems he faces to being labelled as handicapped, not to his personal limitations, whatever they may be. He would perhaps agree with the view that his disability is socially created, and that he is experiencing 'socially imposed restriction' (French, 1993a:19). In this chapter I explore the implications of applying a model of disability as socially imposed restriction to people with learning disabilities. People with learning disabilities have not always been seen as 'disabled'. We can see this reflected in the ongoing debate over terminology, what we call people who appear to be less intellectually competent than the norm. In this chapter I use the term 'learning disability' which aligns the problem with disability more generally. But in the past people with learning disabilities have been legislated for as if they have more in common with people who are mentally ill, for example the 1959 Mental Health Act applied to both subnormality and mental illness. The more recently coined term 'people with learning difficulties' places the problem within an educational/psychological framework. By choosing to use the term 'learning disability' I consciously try to integrate the experiences of the people so labelled within the framework of the social model of disability, and to examine the implications of that perspective for practice and research. (see chapter 1 for a full discussion of the social model of disability).

The chapter falls into two parts. In the first part I begin by applying the social model of disability to learning disability, and comparing it to the principle of normalization which has been so influential in shaping policy and practice in the field. I then try to identify some of the processes which have led to the social construction of learning disability, and some of the barriers people with learning disability face in taking control of their own lives. The second part of the chapter examines how two projects have tackled some of the issues which disempower people with learning disabilities, and the strengths and limitations of these approaches. The first project is a self-advocacy conference; the second is an innovative piece of research. In the light of the discussion I conclude with some thoughts on the potential of developing a theoretical perspective on learning disability which aligns it to the broader disability movement.

The social model of disability compared to normalization

This chapter is based on the assumption that the barriers faced by people with learning disabilities are at least in part socially created, rather than solely the result of the individual's intellectual impairment. As Farber put it, the life chances of people with learning disability are determined 'both by being labelled as deviants and by their incompetence' (1968: 19; quoted in Oliver 1990).

The application of the social model to learning disability is a relatively recent development. Throughout the 1980s the theory or principle of normalization was the dominant perspective. The principle of normalization has various differing manifestations (see Emerson, 1992 for a brief history), but for the purposes of this chapter it can be summed up as 'utilisation of means which are as culturally normative as possible in order to establish and/or maintain personal behaviours and characteristics which are as culturally normative as possible'. (Wolfensberger, 1972: 28). As Brown and Smith (1992) observe in introducing their reader on the subject, normalization has as yet made little impact on service delivery in the field of physical disability. The influence of normalization on the field of learning disability is symptomatic of its separation from other disability groups. Normalization has not attracted much attention from disabled academics. Mike Oliver in an important book, *The Politics of Disablement* (1990), makes no analysis of normalization, and though some disabled authors, for example Morris (1993) and French (1993b), discuss and challenge the social assumption that disabled people want to be 'normal', these debates are not directed at the principle of normalization per se.

So, how does normalization differ from the social model of disability as a way of explaining and addressing the situation in which disabled people find themselves? Fiona Williams (1989) answers this question within the framework of oppression. She identifies people with learning disabilities as an oppressed group and outlines three strategies for liberation from oppression. The first of these she describes as 'integration'—mainstream schooling and housing, the rights to a lifestyle enjoyed by the majority. This is the philosophy underpinning normalization. It is represented by the Ordinary Life principles pursued on behalf of people with learning disabilities under the banners of integration and normalization (Kings Fund Centre, 1980). The improvement this brings when compared with what went before must not be underestimated, but the limitations of this approach are that definitions of normality are far from straightforward, and the use of culturally-valued means to achieve culturally-valued ends as advocated by Wolfensberger may actually reproduce discrimination, on grounds of gender, race, sexual orientation, age etc. (Smith and Brown, 1989; Ferns, 1992). Assumptions are made about what 'devalued people' want as a group, and their voices as individuals are relatively unimportant.

Williams' second form of resistance to oppression, withdrawal from the world into self-contained communities with their own sets of values need not detain us long here, though it has its advocates, for example L'Arche communities. The third of these strategies for resistance is the formation of autonomous groups in which oppressed people—women, black people, disabled people—can raise their consciousness and develop their own analysis of their situation as a means of empowerment. Ultimately, this strategy requires intervention in the institutions of society in order to change them. It recognizes that there are conflicts of interest between providers of services and oppressed groups, and that, if things are to change, disabled people must begin to impose their own values and definitions.

In summary, then, the principle of normalization proposes that disabled people should be enabled to enter the world as it is, and enjoy the rights most people enjoy, but the onus is on them to conform, and on services to enable them to do so. The focus of implementors and interpreters of normalization has been to enhance the lives of devalued individuals rather than change the processes of valuation and devaluation (Novack Amado, 1988: 303). Within the social model, by contrast 'people become disabled only when their society is unable or unwilling to incorporate them and takes steps to marginalise and disempower them on the basis of impairment' (Chappell, 1992: 44). In this scenario it is society which is required to change, not individuals.

The social construction of learning disability

Mike Oliver (1990) makes the point that disability is not an absolute but varies from culture to culture. In a rare attempt to develop cross-cultural perspectives on what he calls mental retardation, Edgerton asks why some cultures regard it as 'seriously troublesome and other do not' (1976: 63). In fact, the history of learning disability, like the history of disability more generally, is exceedingly little researched (Oliver, 1990; Thomson, 1992), and it is largely a matter of speculation rather than scholarship to answer Edgerton's important question in relation to contemporary western societies. Some authors, notably Ryan and Thomas (1987) and Oliver (1990) argue that it was the introduction of factory-based work during the Industrial Revolution which led to disabled people being singled out as deviants requiring specialist facilities and medical treatment. The increasing importance of time keeping, maintenance of production norms, and, later, literacy and numeracy, meant people who had once found an economically useful niche in domestic-scale economic units no longer had a socially productive role.

Specifically in relation to learning disability we can surmise that in societies where literacy was uncommon, people who were unable to read and write did not stand out as they do today. The introduction of education for all in the late nineteenth century in Britain brought the 'problem' of 'feeble-minded' children to public attention; 'with no compulsion for children to be kept at school those who "did not get on well" would have been quietly withdrawn by parents who saw other uses for money laid out in school pence' (Hurt, 1988: 123). Once schooling was made compulsory in 1876 those children who did not profit from education became increasingly hard to ignore, and there was a proliferation of special classes, reports and pseudo-scientific classifications in the period 1882 to 1914 (Hurt, 1988: chapters 5 and 6). Economic conditions also bear on the social construction of learning disability. Employability of people who are intellectually slow depends in part on the state of the job market; during and immediately after the Second World War labour shortages led to the employment of approximately half a million disabled people, including people with learning disabilities, who had hitherto been classified as unemployable (Humphries and Gordon, 1992).

The debate over terminology reflects the difficulties in defining learning disability. Roughly 2 to 3 per cent of the population in western societies are labelled as having learning disabilities (Jenkins, 1993), but less than a third of these have an identifiable organic pathology such as Down's Syndrome. The classification of the rest seems to depend on assessment based on IQ 'and whose deficiency is considered by expert opinion to be severe enough or sufficiently troublesome to others to require special identification' (Jenkins, 1993). It is possible to recognize here the 'medical model' in which disability is defined as a problem inherent in the individual, to be classified and diagnosed by professionals. Social competence appears to be a factor: 'In the absence of a specific impairment it is not usually enough to simply have a low IQ or poor intellectual functioning to be categorised as mentally handicapped' (Jenkins, 1991). Moreover, there is a tendency for mild learning disability to be associated with low social class—'mild mental retardation mainly occurs in families in which the father has an unskilled or semi skilled manual job' (Rutter and Madge, 1976)—and with age: there are proportionately more people defined as having learning disabilities of school age than there are adults, suggesting that the educational system highlights people's intellectual shortcomings which may not be such significant factors in successful functioning in adult life (Tomlinson, 1985).

Although defining 'learning disability' is difficult, the consequences for people who are so labelled are far reaching, and are not dissimilar to those experienced by other disabled people. The majority do not enter the job market, and spend their adult lives in special institutions where they interact primarily with other disabled people, and staff paid to care for them. In common with others who are reliant on State benefits, incomes are low, and poverty is a barrier to full participation in society. This is exacerbated by a benefits system which confines people to a marginal place in the labour market. There is no sliding scale of benefits for people who are construed as dependent as a result of disability, and if employment is accepted people lose their entitlement to disability-related benefits: Brian, interviewed in my recent research (Walmsley, forthcoming), told me he could not convert his part-time job at a Garden Centre (paying him £12 for a three-day week) to full-time employment because his family dare not risk his becoming liable for poll tax, and losing his 'pension'.

The impact this has on people's sense of themselves is hard to quantify. Atkinson and Williams argue that the accounts in their anthology 'point, on the one hand to a very fragile and tenuous link with the conventional forces that shape and reinforce adult identity—paid work, parenthood, leisure pursuits. On the other hand they indicate a very tenacious hold on a sense of self' (1990: 243). The point is well made by Colin, one of the contributors:

> I went to a school for special needs . . . for people who didn't get on with other people. I didn't know why I went there, it was never explained to me. I don't know how my mum felt about it, I never asked her. I never asked anybody except one teacher who said it was because I didn't get on with anybody which wasn't true. (1990: 156).

Colin's analysis is particularly interesting because he demonstrates how hard it is for people to make sense of their experiences in isolation. In some respects, the commitment to normalization has discouraged people from getting together to develop understanding, for, if the most valued relationships are with non-disabled people, then relationships with other disabled people are undesirable. 'If they are discouraged from associating, how can they develop a collective response to discrimination?' (Chappell, 1992: 45).

Agendas for change

The preceding section has begun to outline some of the barriers facing people with learning disabilities in taking greater control of their lives. Current policy can be seen very much within a normalization framework. The emphasis is on gaining access to what have variously been called 'patterns of life . . . which are as close as possible to the regular circumstances and ways of life of society' (Nirje, 1976), 'an ordinary life' (Kings Fund Centre, 1980) or 'valued social roles' (Wolfensberger and Thomas, 1983). Self-advocates at the Third International People First Conference held in Canada at the time this was written (July 1993) summed up what they want in three words: 'integration' (in real homes in the community); 'productivity' (in real jobs paying proper wages), and 'inclusion' (in mainstream services and facilities) (Booth and Booth, 1993a). Official government policy now espouses the principle that people should be helped 'to lead, as far as possible, full and independent lives' and that services for people with learning disabilities should be provided with 'proper participation of the individuals concerned' (HMSO, 1989). Professionals are now expected to facilitate this. This marks a major landmark in intention. But the agendas for change, if the oppression of people on the basis of learning disability is to cease, are huge. 'A society which valued people with learning difficulties would have to question seriously the primacy it gives to cognitive skills at the expense of other attributes, such as emotional wisdom, insight and imagination. In turn it would have to examine the institutions of education, paid work and financial rewards which sustain these priorities' (Williams, 1989: 259). With such an agenda, where do you start?

Self advocacy: spreading the word

Work in groups can enable people to articulate the commonality of their oppression and begin to develop their own agendas for change. Self advocacy is now well developed in Britain, and groups such as People First, Skills for People and Nottingham Advocacy in

Action are established and respected self-advocacy organizations independent of services, and which, at least to some extent, generate their own income through training, consultancy and publications. However, as with other 'new social movements' the members of these groups represent an elite who, through their involvement with self advocacy have developed skills, confidence and understanding which can set them apart from the mass of people with learning disabilities—when I visited People First in London they were waging their own internal campaign against jargon!

Women First 1992

In order to spread the message of self advocacy, and to establish new groups, some self-advocacy organizations run conferences. One such event was the Women First Conference held in Nottingham in 1992 (for a full account see Walmsley, 1993). This was an attempt to allow the voices of women with learning disabilities to be heard. Women in other walks of life have the opportunity to debate women's issues; why not women with learning disabilities? One of the strengths of the conference was an emphasis on it being an opportunity for women with learning disabilities to share experiences with one another, and see women like themselves taking a lead role. The organization of the conference was undertaken by Nottingham Advocacy in Action, run by disabled co-workers, and several non-disabled women. Considerable efforts were made to ensure that women with learning disabilities were involved in the planning, were in the majority at the conference, had leading roles as workshop leaders, and could afford to come. The day was a great success. Over two hundred women came, met one another, shared ideas, feelings, experiences, food. Many evaluated the event positively: for example, 'It was really fun meeting a new group, it was really fun travelling to Nottingham'. 'This was the first conference we had ever been to.' At one workshop forty women addressed together the experience of being abused. For some it was the first time they had acknowledged it. One wrote; 'I found the abuse very interesting. I have been through it.'

Events such as these can be very powerful. They provide rare opportunities to meet others, swap stories, develop understanding and solidarity, all important prerequisites for those women to take charge of their own lives, and begin to articulate what they want for themselves. And yet there are limitations. How do you sustain the momentum?

The follow up to the conference shows that the structures to sustain self advocacy are fragile indeed. Many women went away intending to keep contact and start their own women's groups. Yet this has not happened to any great extent. The creation of such networks requires funding for people to attend meetings, communication without relying on traditional means such as written newsletters, minutes, phone calls and faxes, finding sympathetic allies for transport, particularly in rural areas, or where the streets do not feel safe, or for people who are not able to use public transport. The barriers became obvious when I invited some conference goers to come to talk to a group of women practitioners and academics about Women First. We offered expenses, but had to rely, not on the enthusiasm of the delegates, but on service providers to provide transport. It was the service providers who answered the phone, not women with learning disabilities. In the end, it was the goodwill of women without learning disabilities which had made Women First possible, and one conference was not enough to challenge the powerlessness and the poverty which are the lot of most people with learning disabilities. Days like Women First are important. They offer a vision of how things might be. But they also highlight just how many barriers inhibit women with learning disabilities from taking control.

Research in partnership

Research which involves people with learning disability as partners is rare indeed. It would not be too far fetched to claim that only since the mid 1980s have researchers seriously tried to use people's own accounts as a means of describing the lives, hopes and aspirations of people with learning disabilities. One example of excellent partnership research which seeks to elicit the views of people with learning disabilities is described here. It breaks new ground and sets ethical standards which deserve a wide audience.

Listening to parents

Tim and Wendy Booths' study, funded by the Nuffield Foundation, seeks to make good deficiencies in research on parents with learning disabilities, which they say 'has been conducted from a clinical, developmental or behavioural perspective which has tended to treat the parents as little more than dependent variables in the analysis rather than credit them with any integrity as people' (Booth and Booth, forthcoming). The views of parents in their study are given 'pride of place'; two principles are clearly enunciated:

1. People with learning disabilities are people first, and have the same value, rights and responsibilities as other adults.

2. The researcher treats the interests of the research subject as if they were the researcher's own, ie the commitment is first to the welfare of the parents and their children, not the research.

In pursuing the research the Booths located informants through carefully briefed intermediaries (usually workers) who knew the parents, and who, after explaining the research to them, asked permission to release their names and addresses to the research team. In this way, the pitfall of assuming people with learning disabilities were 'research fodder' was avoided—although it is interesting that 'normal' research approaches, by letter, or asking for volunteers in newspapers or magazines, were not applicable because few could read, and only a handful regularly bought magazines or newspapers.

Permission received, and introductions made, the research proceeded in what the researchers term a 'naturalistic' way. The parents were allowed to dictate the pace—no pre-set questions or time limits—and as many meetings as were mutually deemed useful were held. Usually meetings were on the parents' home territory, and tape recorded, though only with permission. The researchers note wryly the tendency to disclose sensitive information only after the tape recorder was switched off, and are emphatic that note taking during an interview should be avoided, except where absolutely vital. If people cannot read, making notes on them can seem a highly threatening activity, one reminiscent of controlling professional/client interactions, and unlikely to encourage disclosure. The researchers cite instances of the success of their careful approach by reference to the trust some parents felt in them; people would telephone to ask when they would next meet, and ask the researcher to accompany them on a stressful occasion, such as a court appearance.

The importance of such research is indicated by the type of insights gained into people's perceptions of the professional help they were offered. Julie and Neville have a son, Jeremy, who was 18 months old at the time of the research. They lived on a run-down council estate, and were visited by five different workers during the course of a week. The researchers write:

> All visits were recorded in a book kept in the living room. The entries were often derogatory in tone and praiseworthy comments were rare: for example, 'Julie was in a bad mood today and I had to tell her off for not hoovering the carpet.' Julie and Neville cannot read and the book annoyed them intensely: 'If they keep writing in that book I'm going to put it at the back of the fire. They're not me mum to make me do.'

The couple felt confused, angry and fearful about the contacts they had with professionals. Having had their first child taken from them, they were terrified that Jeremy too would be removed if they did not live up to the standards expected: 'Her [Julie's] sister reinforced the point: Sometimes they say to her, "Your baby's not clean enough. If you don't clean him up we'll have to take him off you" ' (Booth and Booth, 1993b).

The written accounts of the research were produced in partnership with the research 'subjects'. They were encouraged to comment on the way they were represented, the choice of extracts and the conclusions. Stories like Julie and Neville's became a basis from which to draw out practice implications, in particular the importance of recognizing that people's difficulties with parenting may not be solely due to individual deficit, and as much or more caused by environmental stresses (poor housing, poverty), absence of good models of parenting, social isolation, inappropriate and unsympathetic professional support, and a tendency on the part of others to believe that parents with learning disabilities will not make good parents. This is in sharp contrast to previous studies of parents which have examined in detail their individual deficits without recognizing the genuine material constraints under which they operate.

The value of studies such as this is that they can frame a set of 'good practice principles grounded on parents' perceptions of their own needs for the guidance of service providers and practitioners.' (Booth and Booth, 1993b). In a practical way, they give a voice to people with learning disabilities where there was none before.

The strengths of this research are that it takes people with learning disabilities seriously, and accords value to their views and experiences. However, it is also important to recognize that it is within a framework where people with learning disabilities remain the junior partners. It was not their research; it was initiated, funded and sustained by others. It is difficult in present circumstances to imagine it being otherwise. The 'material relations of research production' as Zarb (1992) terms them are such that neither researchers nor disabled people are in control, but funding bodies and policy makers. Zarb argues for 'emancipatory research' which is undertaken by, with and for disabled people, and is characterized by 'reciprocity' and 'empowerment'. Imagine for a moment what this may have looked like. Perhaps a group of parents with learning disabilities getting together, deciding that they wanted to find out more about why people like them were having such a hard time, raising some money, employing interviewers, or doing it themselves, supervising the production of the report, and finding someone to publish it. It is almost impossible to visualize such a scenario given the way things are at present; yet it is such a vision that application of the social model of disability can create. The type of approach adopted by the Booths is an important step in recasting the agenda of research so that people with learning disabilities are seen as partners, not 'subjects' but there is a long way to go before such research is actually initiated and controlled by people with learning disabilities. (I am grateful to the Booths for allowing me to see drafts of their forthcoming book to be published by Open University Press). (For further details of emancipatory research, readers are referred to chapter 10.)

Conclusion

In this chapter I set out to apply some of the analyses and critiques developed in relation to disability to the situation of people with learning disabilities. Whilst recognizing that each group has its own history, social issues, ideologies and subjective experiences (Williams, 1989), I argued that an analysis which identifies disability as socially imposed restriction has as much to offer as the influential principle of normalization, which puts the onus to change on individuals rather than on social institutions. There are differences, however. One of these is that though I have quoted the written views of disabled academics—Jenny Morris, Sally French, Mike Oliver—I have not been able to draw on such a rich vein of analysis by people with learning disabilities. Most disabled people could read and understand this paper. It is unlikely that many people with learning disabilities could do so in its present form. This is not to say that people with learning disabilities have not analysed their situation; indeed, I have quoted several who have. But it is to acknowledge that the written word, powerful as it is to communicate and develop ideas, is a medium which excludes people with learning disabilities as effectively as steps exclude people in wheelchairs from buildings. It is a barrier which can, with help and imagination, be overcome, just as steps can be surmounted or replaced. But it is an important difference that serves to emphasize that the interests and needs of different groups do not necessarily coincide, and may indeed conflict. What disabled people do have in common is important; but their differences must not be ignored.

On a more positive note the two examples cited here are not isolated ones. There are a wealth of exciting and imaginative developments I could have chosen to illustrate how people with learning disabilities, and people allied with them, are struggling to find ways forward. They show how people with learning disabilities can be involved in setting principles for practice, in training, in conferences and in developing a collective voice. This is not to deny the power of the structural factors which exclude people from integration, productivity and inclusion; but it is to suggest that taking a social model and applying it to learning disability may offer as much prospect of change as attempting to normalize people so they can fit more easily into the status quo.

References

Atkinson, D. and Williams, F. (eds) (1990) *Know Me As I Am: An Anthology of Prose, Poetry and Art by People with Learning Difficulties*, Hodder & Stoughton, Sevenoaks.

Booth, W. and Booth, T. (1993a) A celebration of stories. *Community Living*, October

Booth, W. and Booth, T. (1993b) Learning the hard way: practice issues in supporting parents with learning difficulties. *Social Work and Social Sciences Review*, 4 (2)

Booth, W. and Booth, T. (forthcoming) *Parenting under Pressure: Mothers and Fathers with Learning Difficulties*, Open University Press, Buckingham.

Brown, H. and Smith, H. (eds) (1992) *Normalisation: A Reader for the Nineties*, Routledge, London.

Chappell, A. L. (1992) Towards a sociological critique of the normalisation principle. *Disability, Handicap and Society*, 7 (1), 25–51

Edgerton, R. (1976) *Deviance: a Cross Cultural Perspective*, Benjamin/Cummings, London.

Emerson, E. (1992) What is normalisation? In *Normalisation: A Reader for the Nineties* (eds H. Brown and H. Smith), Routledge, London.

Farber, B. (1968) *Mental Retardation: Its Social Context and Social Consequences*, Houghton Mifflin, Boston.

Ferns, P. (1992) Promoting race equality through normalisation. In *Normalisation: A Reader for the Nineties* (eds H. Brown and H. Smith), Routledge, London.

French, S. (1993a) Disability, impairment, or something in between? In *Disabling Barriers—Enabling Environments*, (eds J. Swain, V. Finkelstein, S. French and M. Oliver) Sage, London.

French, S (1993b) Can you see the rainbow? The roots of denial. In *Disabling Barriers—Enabling Environments* (eds J. Swain, V. Finkelstein, S. French and M. Oliver) Sage, London.

HMSO (1989) *Caring for People: Community Care in the Next Decade and Beyond*. Cm. 849, HMSO, London.

Humphries, S. and Gordon, P. (1992) *Out of Sight: The Experience of Disability 1900–1950* Northcote House, Plymouth.

Hurt, J. (1988) *Outside the Mainstream: A History of Special Education* Batsford, Oxford.

Jenkins, R. (1991) Disability, and social stratification. *British Journal of Sociology*, 42 (4), 557–580

Jenkins, R. (1993) Incompetence and learning difficulties: anthropological perspectives. *Anthropology Today*, **9 (3)**, 16–20

Kings Fund Centre (1980) *An Ordinary Life*, Kings Fund Centre, London.

Morris, J. (1993) Gender and disability. In *Disabling Barriers—Enabling Environments* (eds J. Swain, V. Finkelstein, S. French and M. Oliver), Sage, London.

Nirje, B. (1976) The normalisation principle. In *Changing Patterns in Residential Services for the Mentally Retarded* (eds R. Kugel and A. Shearer), President's Committee on Mental Retardation, Washington DC

Novak Amado, A. R. (1988) A perspective on the present and notes for new directions. In *Integration of Developmentally Disabled Individuals into the Community*, (2nd edn) (eds L. W. Heal, J. I. Haney and A. R. Novak Amado), Paul H. Brookes, Baltimore, Maryland.

Oliver, M. (1990) *The Politics of Disablement*, Macmillan, London.

Oliver, M. (1992) Changing the social relations of research production? *Disability, Handicap and Society*, **7 (2)**, 101–114

Rutter, M. and Madge, N. (1976) *Cycles of Disadvantage* Heinemann, London, 110.

Ryan, J. with Thomas, F. (1987) *The Politics of Mental Handicap*, Free Association Books, London

Smith, H. and Brown, H. (1989) Whose community: whose care? In *Making Connections* (eds A. Brechin and J. Walmsley), Hodder & Stoughton, Sevenoaks.

Thomson, M. (1992) *The Problem of Mental Deficiency in England and Wales c. 1913–1946*. Unpublished PhD thesis, University of Oxford, Oxford.

Walmsley, J. (1993) Women first: lessons in participation. *Critical Social Policy*, **38** 86–99.

Walmsley, J. (forthcoming) *Gender, caring and learning disability*, Unpublished doctoral research, Open University, Milton Keynes.

Williams, F. (1989) Mental Handicap and oppression. In *Making Connections* (eds A. Brechin and J. Walmsley), Hodder & Stoughton, Sevenoaks.

Wolfensberger, W. and Tullman, S. (1982) A brief outline of the principal of normalisation. *Rehabilitation Psychology* **27**, 131–145

Wolfensberger, W. (1983) Social role valorisation: a proposed new term for the principle of normalisation. *Mental Retardation* **21**, 234–9

Zarb, G. (1992) On the road to Damascus: first steps towards changing the relations of disability research production. *Disability, Handicap and Society*, **7 (2)**, 125–138

12

Families in transition

John Swain and Carole Thirlaway

Understanding 'family transitions'

In this chapter disability will be viewed from the perspective of the family. We have chosen to focus in particular on disabled adolescents and young adults, of an age span roughly between 10 and mid-20s, and their families. We will also concentrate on young people with learning difficulties, though we believe that the issues will have wider application to young disabled people generally. To help us in the enterprise we conducted a small-scale study involving interviews with twelve participants (young people, parents, siblings, a physiotherapist and a community nurse) in a school for young people with learning difficulties. We also drew on a transcript of an interview we conducted with Jean and Norman Willson, the parents of Vicky, a 22-year-old woman with Tuberous Scoliosis. This is not, however, a report of the research, but we shall use quotes from the interviews to illustrate and illuminate our discussions.

In this opening section we give our reasons for our particular focus and, in doing so, provide an overview of the perspective we are taking and introduce the main issues which we shall be discussing in this chapter.

A community nurse told us:

> Well it's got to be one of the two most difficult areas. The other is when they are very young and the parents are first coming to terms with it. Then they seem to get into it to varying degrees, and then suddenly young adolescence is another stage and families have to cope with the change from childhood to adulthood.

This is, indeed, a highly significant period for all concerned. There is evidence that the passage into adulthood can be one of the most stressful periods for families in general (Olsen et al., 1983). For families with young people with learning difficulties this period, as the community nurse suggests, can take on a particular significance. Jean Willson told us:

I think those things, the transition, were mind-boggling. . . . She's got friends the same age, and I know they all experience the same things, you know, because it's like . . . well it's like looking at their childhood and the door closes. And you say, what childhood? Where did it go? And unlike my other daughter and other people's sons and daughters, you are full of hope and expectation, because usually they are going to fly the nest. They are going to go on to university, or they are going to get a job. They're going to leave home, and you've done a good job. Right. Your role is being affirmed for you. There they are. They are going, and I'm pleased to let them go.

I found her 18th birthday and her 21st birthday extremely difficult. On the one hand you want to celebrate the life, and everybody's saying 'yeah we're feeling really happy.' And the other feeling is, what life? What are we celebrating? What on earth do we give to you? And all through her childhood we haven't looked towards her future because it's looked so bleak. What is there? We know there isn't going to be anything when she leaves school. There's nothing. There's a huge empty void, and that's terrifying. And living with that fear for a long time, a lot of parents, it traumatises you. You go back in on yourself.

The meaning of this transition reaches into expectations of what is 'normal' and even the meaning of the term 'learning difficulties', particularly with the connotations it can have of 'eternal childhood'.

What, then, is this 'transition' which seems so crucial in our society? The idea of transitions is ostensibly clear when it is seen as a period of change for an individual, from one stage of the life cycle to another. When applied to the period of adolescence, the picture can be simplified with the usual labels, that is a change from childhood to adulthood. The next step in understanding is the description of each stage, so that 'adulthood' or an adult social identity may be characterized as involving leaving the parental home, having an income and developing sexual relationships. This is, however, only one way of looking at this period of transition. It is built on beliefs that there are particular stages in the life cycle and they can be defined in terms of characteristics, events and so on. Behind such definitions lurk assumptions about 'normality'. Is a person who still lives with his or her parents, has no job and no sexual relationships not an adult? And is the reverse necessarily true, that is that a person who has left the parental home and so on is an adult? Do all the criteria need to be fulfilled?

There are other ways of defining adulthood which may also be relevant. For instance, does age alone define adulthood? The notion of 'age-appropriateness' has been developed as a criterion for evaluating services for people with learning difficulties. In this light, people with learning difficulties should be treated as adults even if the usual characteristics of adult social status are not fulfilled. Yet another way to define adulthood is by self-identity. Thus it can be argued that whether people are adults depends very much on whether they see themselves as such. Furthermore, adulthood can be seen as a legal term, that is defined by the legal rights and obligations set down in legislation.

All the above factors do have a bearing in understanding this lengthy and complex period of adolescence. A job, a home, legal status, sexual relationships and so on are symbolic of adult status, but there is something more fundamental which underlies the actual *process* of transition. The key to this was succinctly expressed by a physiotherapist we interviewed: 'I think the biggest difference when children become an adult is the choice that you give them.' The process of transition can be defined essentially as one of emancipation from childhood dependency towards 'the person's participation in determining the direction of his or her life journey' (Cowan, 1991: 8). This depends not just on the individual, but also on the choices and opportunities that are available. Transition represents the interplay between on the one hand, political, social and economic change, and on the other hand, change for the individual. It is a process which will be experienced differently depending on such factors as race, class and disability. Certainly, disabled people experience considerable restrictions and barriers which limit participation in decision-making processes and thus dis-able transition to adulthood.

The picture becomes even more complex when the term 'transitions' is applied to families rather than individuals as we are attempting to do in this chapter. Even the term 'family' is not as easy to define as it might first appear. Though a nuclear family is still the expected norm, the composition of families in our society varies considerably. It is important to adopt a view of families which incorporates not only siblings and grandparents, for instance, but also one-parent families and families of different class and race.

Even if we can agree on what we mean by 'the family', stages of a family cycle are even harder to define than for an individual. Transitions have meaning for 'the family' not just the individual. Changes for the individual can mean the reorganization of roles and relationships within the whole family system. Within this particular period the process of transition, with shifts of control in decision making, hold the potential for disequilibrium and conflict in families.

Finally, in this chapter, we shall be exploring the possible implications for services and interventions. The physiotherapist we interviewed told us: 'And in this area even our service changes, because I only see people up to the age of 19, after that they go through to adult services.' This is a period which can see changes not only within the family, but also in the services received (and not received). The challenge for all professionals is not just to co-ordinate such changes, but to ensure intervention facilitates and does not obstruct the process of transition.

Identity and expectations

Part of the process of family transitions can generally be seen as the reconstruction of 'the view from within' (Cowan, 1991), which includes a changing view of the self, others and, indeed, the social world. Without such changes it would be debatable whether there actually had been a 'transition'. As applied to young disabled people and their families, major questions are raised concerning the perceptions of adult status and what this might mean in relation to 'disability'.

There is evidence that young people with learning difficulties do come to see themselves as adults. In a study of sixty young people with learning difficulties (Davies and Jenkins, 1993) and their families, they nearly all said that they were adults. From their viewpoint, adult status was indicated by such things as having a key to the front door or being able to have a drink in a pub. This was despite the fact that as few as six of these young people were in full-time open or supported employment, very few managed their own money and the majority were living in their parents' home. This raises the question of the identity of young people as disabled adults and, in particular, the meaning of 'disability' associated with this perceived adult status.

Research suggests that many families 'retain an image of themselves and of "normal" family life that somehow transcends their experience and fondly held beliefs of others' (Hughes and May, 1988: 95). One father we interviewed told us:

> We've always tried to treat Susan as normal. There are certain restrictions, but rather than protect her from the world, we've tried to put her out into the world. And because of that we don't really think of her as having any handicaps.

Such 'denials of disability' or 'lack of acceptance' have often been interpreted as pathological emotional responses to 'the unacceptable'. The need for acceptance is a common message to parents of young people with learning difficulties. It can be an ambiguous message, however. From the viewpoint of a parent, Smith states: 'But it is often unclear just what the parent is being asked to accept: the child's strengths? His limitations? His sexuality? His adulthood? Future placement?' (1988: 155).

Writing from the viewpoint of a disabled person, French shows that it is a 'serious mistake' to see denials of disability in a pathological light. She argues that such denials are rational and lists a number of reasons including: 'to avoid other people's anxiety and distress'; 'to avoid other people's disapproval'; and 'to live up to other people's ideas of "normality" ' (1993: 76). French's argument concerns denial by disabled people themselves, but it seems to us that it can be applied to families as a whole.

There is another form of denial of disability which can be seen as directly relevant to the whole notion of adolescent transitions which we are pursuing. There is evidence that parents do not have high expectations about the possibilities open to their son or daughter and generally accept the status quo (Brotherson et al., 1988). In a study of 269 parents, for instance, it was reported that the majority had no ambitions for their son or daughter in terms of improved working conditions, better wages or advancement (Hill et al., 1985). Such limited expectations were apparent in the interviews we conducted. One parent, for instance, told us:

> What we always said from her being born was if she gets a little real monotonous factory job where all she earns is buttons, that'll get her there and back in the taxi even. So long as it's something she wants to do. She gets up, puts a bit of make-up on, goes out, meets some people, it doesn't really matter so long as she's happy with what she's doing.

Whether it is denied or not, family transitions with disabled adolescents are embedded within a wider social context. Family transitions involve 'reorganisation in the relationships between family members and their social networks outside the family' (Cowan, 1991: 18). For young disabled people there are barriers to transition into adulthood: the barriers in a society geared by and for non-disabled people which exclude disabled people from full active citizenship. Barriers curtail participation in decision making and limit possible choices, and they therefore restrict and determine processes of transition.

Choices and decision making

Leaving school and getting a job can be seen as a major factor in attaining adult status. Surveys of the views of people with learning difficulties have consistently shown that even in times of high unemployment open employment has remained an ideal for many. A study in one day centre, for instance, showed that 60 per cent of people with learning difficulties who used the centre saw finding a job as a priority in their lives (King, 1990).

There is much evidence that disabled people face considerable barriers within the labour market. May and Hughes (1988), for example, reviewed the research relating to leavers from all types of special schools. They concluded that they experienced consistently higher unemployment rates, took longer to find a job in the first place, and much of their employment was in marginal, inherently unstable occupations. This seems to be true even when unemployment rates are generally low. When unemployment rates are high the pattern is uneven: some areas of the country and groups, including disabled people, are more affected than others. For most young people with learning difficulties open employment is not considered to be a realistic option.

The expectation for the vast majority of young people with learning difficulties is that they will attend a day centre after leaving school, perhaps after a period in a college of further education. There has been an expansion of places in further education for people with learning difficulties and as such this is a widening of choice in its own right. Nevertheless, in terms of gaining employment, a college of further education is for the vast majority of young people with learning difficulties a temporary substitute for the day centre.

The lack of employment itself limits participation but can also limit other choices for young people, through, for example, money constraints and restricted social contacts. It is for such reasons that Corbett and Barton state: 'The consequent marginalisation of people with learning difficulties impoverishes their experiences of adulthood' (1993: 26). Nevertheless, gaining employment is not the sole component of the transition process, and some would argue that it is not the most important. Jenkins, for instance, states:

> while long-term unemployment does have detrimental effects on young people during transition to adulthood, it does not seem actually to prevent them from becoming adults. Their potential *access* to particular situations and resources—marriage, for example—may be curtailed by economic constraints; their *rights* in those respects, however, remain intact. Adulthood in British society is a robust, if imprecise, identity, of which people can only be deprived by circumstances that undermine its central portfolio of rights and obligations. (1989: 102)

Jenkins then goes on to argue that young people with learning difficulties are denied such rights and obligations and thus deprived of an adult status.

A major area of rights and obligations which involves adult social status in this society is, of course, leaving the family for a new home, new relationships and, for many young people, children of their own. Again the evidence suggests that young people with learning difficulties face considerable barriers in this transition to adulthood. First, there are barriers to personal relationships outside the family, including lack of money, lack of opportunities, lack of access to leisure activities, lack of self-confidence and lack of awareness (on both sides) (Richardson and Richie, 1989). A recent study of sixty young people found that the social lives of most were closely bound up with those of their parents (Davies and Jenkins, 1993).

The topic of parenting has come to the fore with people moving into the community and also with general changes in attitudes. In this particular arena, however, attitudes can be slow to change (Painz, 1993). For some parents of young people with learning difficulties the idea of their children becoming parents is inconceivable. Talking about sexual relationships, one parent of a young woman with Down's Syndrome told us:

> It's a difficult question. I personally don't have problems with Susan having a sexual relationship. But if that's going to happen then we as parents have to make sure that the idea of contraception's got to be looked at and the only way you can do it, to be absolutely certain, is sterilisation.

Her father went on to say that, 'and the idea of Susan actually going through a wedding ceremony is difficult to comprehend because I don't think she would understand what she was saying.'

Nevertheless, in one of the few studies of parents with learning difficulties, Tim and Wendy Booth found that they 'show more similarities than differences with ordinary families' (1992: 17). They found that the problems parents with learning difficulties faced were mainly to do with lack of money, poor housing, harassment and lack of support. Yet the major cause of upset and trouble for the parents was the attitudes of others, including professionals. 'They're to help you, not to shout at you', said one mother with learning difficulties who had faced opposition from professionals when she decided to get married. Her husband said, 'No one can tell me that a person like Jane isn't the marrying type. You've to live with a person before you can experience it. She's a lovable woman, she's a person you could love. Well, I have done up to 30-odd years. The point is with Jane, you've got to show her the respect' (Swain, 1993: 38–39).

For many people a most significant part of the process of transition to adulthood is the leaving of the parental home. This process is essentially one of young people establishing control over all the day-to-day decisions. The front-door key is symbolic of control by young people over when they come in and go out. It also stands for responsibilities for the security of property. 'Independent living' in the sense that 'independent people' have control over their own lives, not that they perform every task themselves, has been a central element of the disability movement (Brisenden, 1989; French, 1993). Disabled people have sought control over their daily lives. Morris states:

> Control over personal assistance is necessary if those who need help with physical tasks are to achieve both human and civil rights, in other words not only the right to have control over basic daily living tasks (such as when to get up, go to bed, go to the toilet, when and what to

eat) but also the right to have personal relationships, to seek employment, to engage in leisure and political activities. (1993: 8)

While this can also be the ideal for some parents of young people with
learning difficulties, they are often seeking a far more sheltered type
of environment. Susan's father told us: 'I don't think Susan could do
that. I'd hate to put her in a situation where she's the sole manager of
her own time.'

Respite care can be seen as a natural progression towards independent living, parallel to going to stay with friends, going to college
and so on. Seen in this light 'respite' care does not have the negative
connotations of parents 'being unable to cope'. It can provide
opportunities to be with peers and to do things together such as
going to discos and out for a drink. It can also give parents the
opportunity to renew their relationship and spend time with each
other (Oswin, 1984) as other parents can do when their children
reach adulthood.

Transforming family relationships

We now turn to the question: what happens to relationships within
the family through this period of transition? As we have seen the
whole process can differ dramatically when the young person concerned has learning difficulties. The barriers are such that the expected changes may not occur. As Williams and Walmsley say, 'they
may not change their place of residence; they may not change their
social roles; they may not enjoy an enhancement of social status' (1990:
19). The question then has to be translated: what happens to relationships within the family when transitions, or at least the expected
events of transition, do not happen?

The first thing to say about this question is that it brings into public
scrutiny what is usually private. The question can in itself be an
intrusion. Corbett and Barton discuss this issue: 'It is this power to
conflate the public and private spheres and make them the legitimate
concern of professional judgement which demonstrates the degree of
exposure which disabled people have to endure' (1993). Families can
share this exposure and this often involves their experiences being
explained in terms of supposed personal inadequacies. Parents in
their relationship with their son or daughter are in danger of being
seen as over-protective or as being unable to cope with the stress they
are presumed to be under.

From the parents' viewpoint, the transition to adulthood can be a
process of 'letting go'. Jean Willson spoke passionately about the
difficulties they had experienced:

I think the milestone of having a child go through childhood to adulthood and all that means for somebody from the parents' point of view is something you might think, oh god it's going to be a bit heavy, but it was really. . . . And actually recognising her as a woman, and she has a woman's needs not a child's needs. And actually letting go. When she was 18 we said we're going to let go, and we had a plan. But it's one thing to do it and another thing to cope with the feelings.

Other parents have similar feelings. Martin's mother said,

If you have a child you have to let go, don't you? It's very tough if you can't. A measure of your love if you let them go, but it isn't easy. Believe you me, it isn't. It's very difficult. (Richardson, 1989: 8)

The pressures can be experienced by young people as well as parents. One young person with learning difficulties told us: 'They don't want me to leave home at all. My dad goes away and that and my mum gets lonely, so I can never leave home.' The difficulties of letting go, however, are not pathological. Like denials of disability, they are rooted in the experiences, reasoning and feelings of parents. Martin's mother gave two major reasons for the difficulty. The first was the quality of life on offer for her son when he left his parents' home:

He went to a home . . . and when we went to collect him, I cried all the way home. I despaired, because I thought, what's going to happen to my child when I go? He was unkempt, the clothes I had sent I knew had never been worn. . . . I thought, God, I would rather take my child's life—I really mean this, I felt so strongly—than let him go into a place like that. (8)

The second was her whole relationship with her son:

Actually I needed Martin more, to be honest. I only realised it later. I could see that I needed Martin more than he needed me. And if you are honest about it, you do as you get older. You need someone. I'm a touching person, I missed contact. I could cuddle Martin. He didn't like it much but I'd kiss the back of his neck. So I missed this very vital thing for me—the touch. (9)

Susan's mother had similar feelings. Also, like Martin's mother, she felt that Susan was simply not ready for adulthood:

I'm firstly protective because I'm a mother anyway, no matter what she was I wouldn't like it. But there again the other side of me says don't be so daft, you've always let her lead as normal a life as she can. . . . She's never really grown much in the last years so I still see her as a little girl and imagine her in bed with a boy! I can't grasp that. She's still little.

These concerns about letting go can be associated with concerns about the long-term future and all the eventualities, including the death of the parents. The Willsons explained:

> You have to set the wheels in motion and ensure that her needs will be met with or without you, and we're still struggling with this. We've left a will, not that we have a lot of money. I want to make sure people are involved with her life that will help make decisions on her behalf. We've put some money in a trust. It's a small amount of money, but it just gives you a bit of peace of mind.

Other members of the family can be involved in such considerations of the future. There has been a good deal of evidence to show that siblings, especially older sisters, contribute to the care of children with learning difficulties (Stoneman et al., 1988). It would not be surprising then if siblings played a part in plans for securing the future. For some parents it is important that responsibilities will not be forced onto siblings. Again the Willsons explain:

> To be an advocate requires a lot of commitment, to be there every time they're needed. That is a big thing. And we've made it quite clear to our other daughter that she doesn't have to do this at all. We don't expect her, when we turn our toes up, to take over Victoria's care.

Some brothers and sisters, however, take it as a matter of course that their lives can be affected. For instance, talking about why she had chosen to attend a local university, the sister of one young man with learning difficulties told us: 'I've never known any other way of doing things. . . . If I disappear out of his life for six weeks he's going to wonder where I am.' The parents of one young man with learning difficulties spoke to us about the feelings and involvement of their parents. 'People forget about the effect upon grandparents,' they told us. They suggested that family transitions could be doubly difficult for grandparents as they are concerned both for the young people themselves and for the parents.

Services and intervening in family transition

One major factor within the period of transition for families with a disabled adolescent is the changes in services. Many families have grown accustomed to services being co-ordinated and provided within schools and are not prepared to be responsible for locating, acquiring and co-ordinating adult services (Brotherson et al., 1988). For the Willsons this was crucial:

> *Jean*: One of the biggest things is transition from school to nothing. I mean, for us and for Victoria, from school to adulthood filled us with terror, absolute terror. She was going to lose all power, all the input from the school.
> *Norman*: You have to re-establish all the links, only this time you have to do it. There's nobody else.

Jean: But the biggest thing, you see, is that suddenly not only are you going to lose all that, but suddenly your child is an adult, and you lose any power, or you potentially lose any power, because they are deemed as an adult. So suddenly in the eyes of the law, you're not responsible for them.

Norman: They are responsible for themselves.

Jean: It's an absolute nightmare. I mean, to give you a classic example, if for some reason some doctor somewhere decided she ought to have an operation, or her drugs should be changed to a cheaper sort of drugs, you have to fight very hard and be very confident that you are acting as her representative. I mean, you've heard all these cases about sterilization. It's a mine-field with somebody like Victoria. You have to set the wheels in motion and ensure that her needs will be met with or without you.

Much thinking about intervention is rooted in a personal inadequacies model of the family. Utilizing 'the family stress theory', for instance, Tasch makes many recommendations about what parents *must* do, such as 'they must come to terms with their adolescent's current level of functioning' (1988: 98). Such approaches would seem to deny rather than promote the decision-making processes within the family.

Rather than taking family dysfunction as the root of understanding, we would like to stress four points. First, families of disabled adolescents have a variety of strengths which may be mobilized for successful coping (Brotherson et al., 1988). Second, adolescence is a period of potential conflict between the views on self-defined needs of adolescents and other members of their families. Third, families are all different. They adapt and find their own particular ways of functioning. Fourth, 'in the area of professional support, parents describe numerous stresses and difficulties when working with professionals. . . . Many parents felt that in planning for their son's or daughter's future, professionals were insensitive, offered little help, did not know about or offer alternatives, and did not speak "English" ' (Brotherson et al., 1988: 166). (Though we agree with the point being made, it has to be said that for some families English is not their first language.)

It is widely accepted that health professionals, particularly perhaps therapists and nurses working in the community, should work in 'partnership' with families (Marsh and Fisher, 1992). We would like to suggest a number of principles for partnerships in fostering the process of transition:

1. Informal transition planning should begin when the young person is aged about 10 and formal transition planning should be in place by the time he or she reaches 16 years of age (McDonald, McKie and Webber, 1991).

2. The young person with learning difficulties (or his or her designated advocate) should participate in all aspects of the planning
   and decision making. The process of transition should open up
   choices and develop opportunities, relationships and patterns of
   living in line with the young person's individual wishes.
3. The family should be involved in the planning from the beginning.
   They should be given every opportunity to participate in the
   decision-making processes.
4. Intervention should help families in their communication and
   decision making. If it is recognized that sometimes there will be a
   conflict between the needs expressed by the young person and
   those expressed by his or her parents, intervention should open up
   discussions rather than deny conflict or impose solutions. This
   may involve providing information about all the possible options.
5. The partnership is with the family as a whole rather than intervention being based on the presumed needs of the young person with
   learning difficulties. The economic, social and recreational needs
   of the entire family are relevant factors in decisions to be taken by
   the family.
6. Finally, partnerships should look towards the nature and organization of services available to families. The partnership should aim
   to increase the array of vocational, residential and social options
   available in the community and to increase the control of families
   in developing these options.

Conclusion: what transitions?

Anita Binns believed 'we should have the same rights as everybody
else.' She said these rights are:

> The right to make your own decisions.
> Right to make your own mistakes.
> Right to vote.
> Right to be treated as a normal human being.
> Right to proper hospital treatment.

Anita came to believe that she should have these rights through her
experiences, as a person with learning difficulties, of having such
rights denied (Swain, 1993: 42). The physiotherapist we interviewed
said that, 'By the time families of children with severe learning
difficulties reach this transition period, I don't think they've got much
hope left.' When opportunities and choices are limited to the extent
that aspirations have been replaced by acceptance, it is legitimate to
ask the question: What transition?

If preparation and support is to extend opportunities and choice, rather than promote acceptance, it has to be founded on partnership and the expressed needs of those involved. McDonald et al. (1991: 106) advise that: 'Transition planning is the shared responsibility of home, school, and adult services.' There are practical questions to be tackled by this planning partnership: living arrangements; continuing education, leisure and work arrangements. The transference of professional provision, including medical reviews, nursing and therapy services can be crucial to these practical concerns. Nevertheless, planning which facilitates the processes of family transition is not just about the practicalities, it is about people making their own decisions and, indeed, having the right to make their own mistakes. It is to this end that parents can 'convey attitudes of love and respect and help their children develop the skills they will need to live in a social world', and nurses and therapists can 'add their knowledge and expertise by providing counselling, education, training and other services' (Tasch, 1988: 107). In this way, transition planning is a process in which families as a whole develop their confidence to address the issues during this complex period.

References

Booth, T. and Booth, W., (1992) An ordinary family life. *Community Care*, 23 April, **912**, 15–17

Brisenden, S., (1989) A charter for personal care. In *Progress*, **16**, Disablement Income Group, London

Brotherson, M. J., Turnbull, A. P., Bronicki, G. J., Houghton, J., Roeder-Gorgon, C., Summers, J. A. and Turnbull, H. R., (1988) Transitions into adulthood: parental planning for sons and daughters with disabilities. *Education and Training in Mental Retardation*, **23 (3)**, 165–174

Corbett, J. and Barton, L., (1993) *A Struggle For Choice: Students with Special Needs in Transition to Adulthood*, Routledge, London

Cowan, P. A., (1991) Individual and family life transitions: a proposal for a new definition. In *Family Transitions*, (eds P. A. Cowan and M. Hetherington), Lawrence Erlbaum Associates, Hillsdale, New Jersey

Davies, C. A. and Jenkins, R., (1993) Young people with learning difficulties making the transition to adulthood. Findings No 35, Joseph Rowntree Foundation

French, S., (1993) 'Can you see the rainbow?' The roots of denial. In *Disabling Barriers—Enabling Environments*, (eds J. Swain, V. Finkelstein, S. French and M. Oliver), Sage, London

Hill, J., Seyfarth, J., Orelove, P., Wehman, P., and Banks, P. D., (1985) Parent/guardian attitudes towards the working conditions of their mentally retarded children. In *Competitive Employment for Persons with Mental Retardation: From Research to Practice*, (eds P. Wehman and J. W. Hill), Virginia Commonwealth University, Richmond VA

Hughes, D. and May, D., (1988) From child to adult: the significance of school-leaving for the families of adolescents with mental handicaps. In *Living with Mental Handicap: Transitions in the Lives of People with Mental Handicap*, (eds G. Horobin and D. May), Jessica Kingsley, London

Jenkins, R., (1989) Barriers to adulthood: long-term unemployment and mental handicap compared. In *Making Connections*, (eds A. Brechin and J. Walmsley), Hodder & Stoughton, London

King, J., (1990) With a little help from my friends. *Community Care*, 8 March, **804**, 20–21

McDonald, L., McKie, F., and Webber, G., (1991) Transition pilot project: implications for adult service providers. *Canadian Journal of Rehabilitation*, **5 (2)**, 107–111

Marsh, P. and Fisher, M., (1992) *Good Intentions: Developing Partnership in Social Services*, Joseph Rowntree Foundation, York

May, D. and Hughes, D., (1988) From handicapped to normal: problems and prospects in the transition from school to adult life. In *Living with Mental Handicap: Transitions in the Lives of People with Mental Handicap*, (eds G. Horobin and D. May), Jessica Kingsley, London

Morris, J., 1993, *Community Care or Independent Living?*, Joseph Rowntree Foundation, York

Olson, D. H., McCubbin, H., Barnes, H., Larsen, A., Muxen, M. and Wilson, M., (1983) *Families: What Makes them Work*, Sage, Beverley Hills

Oswin, M., (1984) *They Keep Going Away*, King's Fund, London

Painz, F., 1993, *Parents with a Learning Disability*, Social Work Monographs, Norwich

Richardson, A., (1989) 'If you love him, let him go'. In *Making Connections*, (eds A. Brechin and J. Walmsley), Hodder & Stoughton, London

Richardson, A. and Ritchie, J., (1989) *Developing Friendships: Enabling People with Learning Difficulties to Make and Maintain Friends*, Policy Studies Institute, London

Stoneman, Z., Brody, G. H., and Davis, C. H., (1988) Childcare responsibilities, peer relations, and sibling conflict: older siblings of mentally retarded children. *American Journal of Mental Retardation*, **93 (2)**, 174–183

Swain, J., (1993) *Working Together for Citizenship*, Update Workbook, P555 Mental Handicap: Patterns for Living, Open University Press, Milton Keynes

Tasch, V., (1988) Parenting the mentally retarded adolescent: a framework for helping families. *Journal of Community Health Nursing*, **5 (2)**, 97–108

Williams, F. and Walmsley, J., (1990) *Transitions and Change*, Workbook 3, K668 Mental Handicap: Changing Perspectives, Open University, Milton Keynes

13

Working with disabled people from minority ethnic groups

Sally French

It has been shown beyond doubt that illness and impairment are positively correlated with low socio-economic status (Whitehead, 1988; Smith and Jacobson, 1988). People from minority ethnic groups are disproportionately represented in this section of society, and thus their level of illness and impairment is higher than that of the majority population. Asian people, for example, have a higher incidence of diabetes (Patel, 1992), Afro-Caribbean people have a higher incidence of stroke, and the babies of women from many minority ethnic groups are smaller than average, predisposing the infants to impairment. There is, however, considerable variation in the level of illness and impairment among the minority ethnic groups, with Afro-Caribbean people being particularly adversely affected (Lonsdale, 1990).

As well as the link with poverty, there are a number of diseases which mainly affect people from specific minority ethnic groups; one of these diseases is sickle-cell anaemia which is transmitted genetically and is confined mainly to Afro-Caribbean people, though the incidence among other groups is rising (Sickle Cell Society, 1990). It is estimated that one in ten people of Afro-Caribbean origin carries the defective gene, and one in four hundred has the disease. There is a higher than average incidence of tuberculosis, rickets and osteomalacia among Asian people (Donovan, 1984) and specific eye conditions, which can lead to severe visual impairment, are more common in some minority ethnic groups than others, for example, diabetic retinopathy is particularly common among Jewish people, and cataracts are prevalent among Asian people (Royal Association of Disability and Rehabilitation (RADAR), undated). Caucasian people are, of course, similarly affected with a high incidence of specific diseases, such as cystic fibrosis and breast cancer, and thus any tendency to view people from minority ethnic groups in terms of 'problems' is unjustified and should be avoided.

This high incidence of illness and impairment is offset by the relatively low percentage of older people from minority ethnic groups in Great Britain, due to the fact that many people emigrated after the Second World War when they were young. In a few years time many will reach old age and their health and social needs will become more urgent.

Despite these variations it must be borne in mind that low socio-economic status, often resulting from racism, and leading to poor housing, diet and unemployment, is far more influential than ethnic origin or cultural difference with regard to the incidence of illness and impairment (Confederation of Indian Organizations, 1987; Smith and Jacobson, 1988). White people have traditionally emphasized cultural differences to explain racial inequalities, thereby avoiding the realities of white domination and power. However, people from minority ethnic groups should not be stereotyped as poor, unemployed and disadvantaged, and the enormous differences in terms of language, religion and social customs between people from different minority ethnic groups should be remembered; they do not form a homogeneous group and the majority population may resemble some minority ethnic groups in terms of culture more than the minority ethnic groups resemble each other.

Services for people with illnesses and impairments specific to their minority ethnic status have been neglected. Grimsley and Bhat (1988) point out that uncommon conditions which affect Caucasian people, such as phenylketonuria, are screened, implying that diseases such as sickle-cell anaemia would be if they affected the majority population. Bryan et al. (1985) and the Sickle Cell Society (1990) point out the general lack of interest in sickle-cell anaemia by health professionals. Tuberculosis, which is also more common in certain minority ethnic groups, has, in contrast, had a high profile, probably because of its threat to the majority population. The lack of knowledge of diseases which specifically affect people from minority ethnic groups can easily interact with racist attitudes concerning illness behaviour, leading to a lack of belief in symptoms, such as pain, of which a person is complaining. This is a common experience of people with sickle-cell anaemia (Sickle Cell Society, 1990). Impairment can also interact with racial stereotyping; people with hearing impairments, for example, may be regarded as illiterate, unable to comprehend English, and stupid (Disability—Identity, Sexuality and Relationships, 1991).

Take up of services

It has frequently been noted that disabled people from minority ethnic groups tend not to use the health and social services which are available, such as meals on wheels, aids and equipment, rehabilitation and preventative medicine (Greater London Association of Disabled

People (GLAD), 1987). The uptake of benefits is also low (Baxter et al., 1990). They are very often blamed for this behaviour, but on close inspection it is not difficult to understand the reasons for it.

Lack of knowledge of services

A general lack of knowledge about what services exist has been found among disabled people from some minority ethnic groups (Confederation of Indian Organizations, 1987; Baxter et al., 1990). This includes lack of awareness of statutory services, aids and equipment, disability organizations, community groups and benefits. There is also uncertainty, particularly among those who do not have British citizenship, regarding their rights, and perhaps a fear of enquiring into such issues too deeply. One of the main reasons for this lack of knowledge is poor provision for people who do not speak English. In addition Jeewa (1990) makes the point that Asian disabled people frequently believe that the services provided are simply not for them. This may, however, be due to the hostility and racism which they have experienced in the past when attempting to use these services (Disability—Identity, Sexuality and Relationships, 1991).

Inappropriate services

Even if disabled people from minority ethnic groups do know of the existence of services, there are a variety of reasons why they may not take advantage of them. When talking of the NHS, Weller states 'this service remains essentially geared to the attitudes, priorities and expectations of the majority population which is considered as white, middle class and nominally Christian' (1991: 31).

An enormous barrier for many disabled people from minority ethnic groups is their inability to speak English very well and the inadequate response of service providers to this difficulty. The resulting lack of communication leads to many serious problems; treatments such as psychotherapy and counselling become impossible and health education becomes inaccessible. Therapists cannot communicate with their patients and clients, and teachers and educational psychologists cannot communicate with disabled children or their parents.

Tomlinson (1990) and Baxter et al. (1990) point out that children whose mother tongue is not English are assessed using tests written in English and may be placed in special schools inappropriately as a result. In addition, developmental tests are culture specific and based on white, middle-class norms which make them even more unsuitable. Crowley (1991) points out that Afro-Caribbean children are over represented in schools for pupils with learning difficulties which may be explained, at least in part, by these cultural biases. On the other hand, any genuine learning difficulties which children from minority ethnic groups have may go undetected or be interpreted as language problems.

With regard to special education, Tomlinson (1990) found that parents of disabled children from minority ethnic groups do not understand the complex assessment and referral procedures, lack knowledge of their parental rights, are confused by receiving conflicting advice from professionals, have problems in keeping in contact with special schools and are dissatisfied with the ethnocentric nature of the curriculum. Some education departments, for example that of the London Borough of Newham, now provide workers from minority ethnic groups to help and befriend parents of disabled children. They also provide literature in many languages giving parents practical advice. A similar scheme also operates in the London Borough of Tower Hamlets (Davis and Choudbury, 1989).

The language problems of deaf and speech-impaired adults and children and their families are compounded as speech therapists rarely operate in languages other than English. There is a need for speech therapists who speak such languages as Punjabi, Gujarati and Urdu (*Therapy Weekly*, 1991). Stokes (1988) states that 20 per cent of people referred to speech therapy in the London Borough of Tower Hamlets are Bengali speakers and that it was impossible to treat them until a Bengali interpreter and assistant were employed.

The problems of communication do, however, run deeper than language. There is a lack of understanding among the majority population concerning the lifestyles, social customs and religious practices of people from minority ethnic groups (Weller, 1991). This can lead to inappropriate service provision. Special bathing aids, for example, may be completely inappropriate for people whose washing methods are different from those of the indigenous population, childcare practices may vary, ways of coping with terminal illness and death may differ (Green, 1989a,b,c,d), and it may be totally unacceptable for people from some minority ethnic groups to be treated by a person of the opposite sex or in view of other patients, in the hydrotherapy pool or gymnasium, for example.

Hospitals, day centres and residential homes are unlikely to attract disabled people from minority ethnic groups unless they provide suitable food, leisure activities, music and religious services; the decor, toys, books and magazines should also reflect the multi-ethnic society in which we live. Even though disabled people and their assistants may be in desperate need of a break from each other, they are unlikely to accept assistance unless it caters for their particular needs. Javed (1993) found that 75 per cent of visually-impaired Asian people surveyed were in favour of a special day centre where their needs as Asian people would be met and respected. As Read reminds us 'In an oppressive society unless you are actively countering the oppression you are perpetuating it. There is no neutral ground' (1988: 14).

Racism, prejudice and stereotyping

Institutional racism can be said to exist when institutions are not geared to meet people's needs and when a uniform culture is assumed (Watkins, 1987). In *Double Bind* (Confederation of Indian Organizations) racism is defined as: 'all attitudes, procedures and practices— social and economic—whose effect, though not necessarily conscious intention, is to create and maintain the power, influence and well being of white people at the expense of black people' (1987: 2). Weller refers to such an attitude as 'ethnocentrism' which she defines as 'the beliefs that the values and practices of one culture are superior or of greater worth than those of an alternative culture' (1991: 31). Hugman (1991) believes that ethnocentric concepts of health underpin professional training. Connelly states that:

> there is little hope that sensitive account will be taken of diversity and the experience of black people when policies, procedures and practices are seen as relatively fixed, when the responsibility of public authorities is seen as provision of standard service on a more-or-less 'take it or leave it' basis, or when it is considered that constrained resources make this the only feasible course. (1988: 10)

For disabled people from the minority ethnic groups, institutional racism is combined with institutional disablism, whereby disabled people are barred from many public buildings and activities because of lack of access or rigid social practices which do not take their needs and rights into account (Hill, 1991). This dual disadvantage subjects people to a great deal of negative discrimination, for example in the employment market. McDonald, who is black and has cerebral palsy, explains, 'to fight for black people is one thing, to fight for the rights of disabled people something else. There is not enough time and energy to fight two different wars' (1991: 8). Similarly Hill states, 'Black disabled people, I have found to my cost, are a discrete minority within a minority' (1990: 45).

There is, at present, very little empirical material on the ways in which race structures the experience of disability (Oliver, 1990), but Stuart (1993) believes that the concept of 'double discrimination' is simplistic, arguing that black disabled people are subjected to a unique type of oppression which is more than the sum of racism and disabilism.

It is the belief of the authors of *Double Bind* (Confederation of Indian Organizations, 1987) that most racism is institutionalized, but that is not to deny that disabled people from minority ethnic groups may experience racist attitudes directly from service providers. Hill states that 'As far as disability is concerned, race and racism is rarely discussed. And all too often providers feel that they do not need to think any more specifically than in terms of disability alone' (1991: 7). Negative attitudes and a lack of understanding of cultural mores and norms of behaviour have led to serious consequences for people from minority ethnic groups, whose behaviour has often been considered odd or mad leading to an over representation of people from certain minority ethnic groups in psychiatric hospitals and hospitals for people with learning difficulties. People from the Caribbean, for example, are much more likely to be diagnosed as schizophrenic and admitted to psychiatric hospitals.

There are different beliefs about health, illness and disability among minority ethnic groups and different ways of responding which health and welfare professionals should understand. For example, Rack (1982) and Crowley (1991) have found that Indian and Pakistani people tend to describe emotional states in terms of physical illness; they may feel it is inappropriate to talk about emotional problems to professionals. There are also cultural differences in people's responses to pain (Melzack and Wall, 1988) though this has probably been exaggerated. To assume that pain and other symptoms are inevitably of psychological origin in members from minority ethnic groups is, however, racist (Ahmad, 1989).

Even pressure groups and organizations such as The British Council of Organizations of Disabled People have been accused of ignoring the needs and rights of disabled people from minority ethnic groups (Hill, 1991), and of a lack of understanding of racism (Disability—Identity, Sexuality and Relationships, 1991). Similarly, those who promote the rights of people from minority ethnic groups have been accused of ignoring disabled people. This situation has given rise to the formation of various groups of disabled people from ethnic minorities, such as the Association of Blind Asians and The Asian People's Disability Alliance. A period of segregation within the disability movement may be necessary in order for disabled people from minority ethnic groups to address and work through the particular issues which concern them.

Service providers often believe that the lack of service uptake among disabled people from minority ethnic groups reflects a greater family and social network than the majority population enjoys. However, this can be used as an excuse for not providing an appropriate

service and has been disputed (Confederation of Indian Organizations, 1987; Baxter et al., 1990, Disability—Identity, Sexuality and
Relationships, 1991; Gunaratnam, 1993). The Greater London Council
of Disabled People (GLAD) (1987) believes that stereotyped beliefs
that Afro-Caribbean people are catered for by their families should be
challenged. For example, GLAD's (1987) report, on a survey in Brent,
revealed that 68 per cent of elderly Afro-Caribbean people live alone.
Similarly McCalman (1990) studied Afro-Caribbean, Asian and
Vietnamese/Chinese carers of old people in the London Borough of
Southwark and found little evidence of an extended family network.

Another common belief among health and welfare professionals is
that the reason for the low uptake of services among disabled people
from ethnic minority groups is their attitude towards disability. For
example, it has been suggested that families can be very protective of
disabled members, leading to lack of opportunity for their disabled
relatives, especially for girls and women, outside the family (Association of Blind Asians, 1990). It has been argued that among Asian
people, disability is sometimes looked upon as shameful or is viewed
as a blessing or as a punishment from God (Baxter et al., 1990). In
Double Bind (Confederation of Indian Organizations) it is stated that,
'Disability is sometimes seen as a "curse" and this can cause the
disabled person, particularly if a woman, to stay hidden away, or even
worse to be hidden away' (1987: 10).

Such feelings and beliefs are not, of course, confined to sections of
the minority ethnic population and may be uncommon among them.
In a study based on twelve Asian families with disabled children
(*Community Care*, 1988) it was found that their attitudes were similar
to those of white families. They were satisfied with their social worker
and were pleased with the summer play schemes arranged for their
children. They would, however, have welcomed the establishment of
an Asian self-help group and special open days for them at the social
service department. The study highlighted a number of misconceptions about Asian families, for example the desire to seek help only
from within the family.

If there is any tendency to keep disability hidden it is certainly
exacerbated by inappropriate services. It is stated in *Double Bind* that:

> Many disabled people now appear to find there is little point in trying
> to obtain benefits. As a consequence this gives the statutory authorities
> and administrators of benefits the excuse to maintain the stereotype of
> either Asian families and communities catering for the needs of their
> own disabled or, even worse, that disabled Asian people do not exist
> or reside in the United Kingdom. (1987: 17)

Simes (1990) believes that Asian people find it difficult to accept that
disability cannot be cured. This is not, of course, uncommon among
the majority population either. Simes states:

> Accepting that the handicap is not an illness but a condition that will last a lifetime is often very difficult for some of the parents. They frequently give for one of their reasons for settling in Britain the hope that because of better medical treatment the child will be cured of the handicap. (1990: 12)

There is also a lack of understanding of the concept of special education among some Asian parents (GLAD, 1987). Tomlinson (1990) believes that the word 'special' is sometimes interpreted as 'good' and 'better than' rather than 'different'. Asian people may assume that because their disabled child is at school, which is viewed as a centre of learning, he or she is capable of academic success. These misconceptions, as well as language barriers, make high quality communication vitally important.

At a more profound level, many beliefs which are shared by the majority population, for example the desirability of independence, may be viewed negatively in cultures which favour collectivism rather than individualism.

This all amounts to a tremendous lack of appropriate services for disabled people from minority ethnic groups, although the situation is slowly improving. Where appropriate services do exist they tend to be found in areas with a high density of people from minority ethnic groups.

What should be done?

Section 20 of the 1976 Race Relations Act makes it unlawful to discriminate against people on racial grounds in terms of facilities, goods and services, the manner in which they are delivered or their quality. Education, high quality management and adequate resources are all necessary if health and caring professionals are to abide by this act.

Race equality training

Health professionals are predominantly white and non-disabled and receive very little training concerning the needs and difficulties of disabled people from ethnic minority groups (Vousden, 1987). It is almost impossible to be entirely free of racist beliefs and attitudes when brought up in a racist society like our own. Some of these attitudes and behaviour patterns may be conscious while others are submerged. It may be that we attend to people from minority ethnic groups a little less than other people, that we do not expect as much of them, or that we give them a little less of our time. In many ways the more subtle and submerged racism becomes the more difficult it is to deal with. Read believes that 'white people have to learn that, although it is not their fault, they are racist, however well intentioned they are, but that they can learn to change their behaviour' (1988: 52).

Race equality training, when skilfully carried out by people from minority ethnic groups, can help us become aware of our attitudes and behaviour in a relaxed and non-threatening environment. Eversley (1989), speaking at a symposium on the health and social needs of people from minority ethnic groups, organized by the College of Occupational Therapists, said that it is no longer acceptable to treat people from minority ethnic groups 'just like everyone else' or to take a 'why can't they be like us?' approach, as this fosters prejudice. The authors of *Double Bind*, talking of Asian disabled people, state that 'True integration is recognising that disabled Asians may have special needs. Treating everyone the same is not equality, because it does not take into account these needs. This would be assimilation and not integration.' (1987: 19).

When considering disabled people from minority ethnic groups, disability equality training is also needed. There are some excellent disability equality training workshops and packs available, which address the issue of race, devised and run by disabled people themselves (Open University, 1990, 1991; London Borough's Disability Resource Team, 1991). Disabled people from minority ethnic groups must be sought and actively involved in the education of health and welfare professionals. (For further information on disability awareness/equality training, the reader is referred to chapter 7).

There also needs to be greater awareness and understanding of the cultural diversity of people from different minority ethnic groups and a sensitivity to these differences when communicating with and treating them. Health and welfare professionals should have a working knowledge of their likely health beliefs, dietary needs, religious practices and social customs, but above all should be prepared to learn from their disabled patients and clients. Attempting to understand cultural differences must not, however, lead to simplification and stereotyping (McGee, 1992). Hugman (1991) believes that cultural knowledge can increase the power of professionals and can be used in a racist way.

Kroll (1990) and Baxter et al. (1990) believe that the training of health professionals fails to prepare them for work in a multi-ethnic society and that an awareness of racism and inequality should be a prominent strand which runs through the curriculum.

Interpreters

There is an urgent need for more trained interpreters. Their shortage is a major problem; in the London Borough of Tower Hamlets, for example, the 1988 census recorded 172 languages (Wilson, 1989). It is common practice in the health service to use relatives of disabled people who cannot speak English as interpreters, including children, which is far from satisfactory. Such people are neither trained nor paid for their services, and their presence may be inappropriate when sensitive information is discussed. In addition child interpreters may not understand the complex issues raised. Watkins believes that it is 'quite inappropriate to expect people to discuss intimate medical problems through their children, relatives or friends' (1987: 207). Disabled people from minority ethnic groups deserve the same confidentiality as everyone else. Baxter et al. (1990) point out that interpreters must be matched carefully to the patient or client; for example, it may be inappropriate for an old person to talk through a young person or someone of the opposite sex.

A register of bilingual staff is helpful and can give rise to a dramatic uptake of services (Baxter, 1988), but Chaudbury believes that interpreters should ideally be independent of the organization. In relation to the education service she states 'Interpreters who see their role as interpreting the LEA's wishes to the parent can very easily slip into putting pressure on to parents to go along with what is being proposed' (1990: 10). Ellis (1993) makes the point that interpreters are frequently used to pass on unpalatable information or to negotiate difficult decisions rather than to facilitate understanding.

It would also be helpful if more written information were translated into minority languages although this should not be regarded as a 'cure all'. Ley (1988) cites evidence, concerning patients and clients generally, that the written word is not always a very effective way of communicating information. Kroll (1990) believes that pamphlets should be used only to consolidate information which has been given orally.

Employment of professionals from minority ethnic groups

In a survey of racial equality in the social services (Commission for Racial Equality) it is stated that 'without equal employment opportunities it is unlikely that there will be equal opportunities in service delivery' (1989: 11). Holden (1988) reports that the social services department of Bradford Metropolitan Council found that the appointment of an Asian worker in a respite team brought a dramatic increase in the number of Asian people using it. In *Double Bind* it is recommended that outreach teams, comprising people from the Asian community, should attempt to reach Asian disabled people and their families who are not using statutory services, to educate them about the services, to befriend them, to act as interpreters, to encourage them to take a more active role in community service and decision-making processes, and to set up their own clubs. They believe that outreach teams should be of the same cultural background as the target groups.

In the programme *Mosaic* (1991) the importance of advocates and initiatives coming from within the minority ethnic communities themselves was stressed. Unfortunately such projects often have great difficulty securing funding and what sometimes happens is that large numbers of people from the particular minority ethnic groups concerned are referred to whatever small facility exists which, as well as overwhelming it, tends to result in less urgency being felt regarding the adaptation of existing mainstream services. It is very important that services are not tokenistic, involving only minor and superficial changes, and that disabled people from minority ethnic groups are not used in a tokenistic way, for example, as sole representatives on committees or in the workforce. Hugman makes the point that equal opportunity policies can serve as a form of image management and that 'Equal opportunity statements can be used as a smokescreen behind which racism remains intact' (1991: 158).

Conclusion

It is clear from the above account that although progress is slowly being made, a great deal still needs to be done to provide disabled people from minority ethnic groups with sensitive and effective health and social services. The attitudes and behaviour of individual practitioners is vitally important in bringing about change, but management backing and the development of policy relating to resources, staff recruitment and working practices must be made at every level of the organization if meaningful progress is to be achieved. Connelly believes that:

> 'Professional' has a number of different meanings. Some are to do with the practice of a particular body of knowledge, but with occupations concerned with social care it is at least as important that the emphasis should be on another meaning; competence—in this case competence in dealing with diversity. Humility and flexibility and willingness to ask questions thus become critical aspects of professional integrity. So too does the strength to take chances, to apply existing and increasing knowledge and skills to new situations. (1988: 2)

References

Ahmad, W. T. U. (1989) Policies, pills and political will: a critique of policies to improve the health status of ethnic minorities. *The Lancet*, **1 (8630)**, 148–150

Association of Blind Asians (1990) London, personal communication

Baxter, C. (1988) *The Black Nurse: An Endangered Species*, National Extension College for Training in Health and Race, London

Baxter, C., Poonia, K., Ward, L. and Nadirshaw, Z. (1990) *Double Discrimination: Issues and Services for People with Learning Difficulties from Black and Ethnic Minority Communities*, King's Fund Centre/Commission for Racial Equality, London

Bryan, D., Denzie, S. and Scafe, S. (1985) *The Heart of the Race: Black Women's Lives in Britain*, Virago, London

Chaudbury, A. (1990) Problems for parents—experiences of Tower Hamlets. In *Asian Children and Special Needs: A Report for ACE*, (ed. C. Orton), Advisory Centre for Education, London

Community Care (1988) Asian families with handicapped children, March 10, 45–46

Confederation of Indian Organizations (1987) *Double Bind: To Be Disabled and Asian*, London

Connelly, N. (1988) *Care in the Multi-racial Community*, Policy Studies Institute, London

CRE (1989) Racial Equality in Social Service Departments, Commission for Racial Equality, London

Crowley, J. (1991) Races apart. *Nursing Times*, **87 (10)**, 44–46

Davis, H. and Choudbury, P. A. (1989) Helping Bangladeshi families: Tower Hamlets Parent Adviser Scheme. In *Making Connections*, (eds A. Brechin and J. Walmsley), Hodder & Stoughton, London

Disability—Identity, Sexuality and Relationships (1991), Video cassette of the Disability Equality Training Pack (K665y), Open University, Milton Keynes

Donavan, J. (1984) Ethnicity and health: a research review. *Social Science and Medicine*, **19 (7)**, 663–670

Ellis, K. (1993) *Squaring the Circle: User and Carer Participation in Needs Assessment*, Joseph Rowntree Foundation, London

Eversley, J. (1989) The same does not mean equal. *Therapy Weekly*, **16 (20)**, 3

GLAD (1987) *Disability and Ethnic Minority Communities—A Study in Three London Boroughs*, Greater London Association of Disabled People, London

Green, J. (1989a) Death with dignity: Islam. *Nursing Times*, **85 (5)**, 56–57

Green, J. (1989b) Death with dignity: Hinduism. *Nursing Times*, **85 (6)**, 50–51

Green, J. (1989c) Death with dignity: Sikhism. *Nursing Times*, **85 (7)**, 56–57

Green, J. (1989d) Death with dignity: Judaism. *Nursing Times*, **85 (8)**, 64–65

Grimsley, M. and Bhat, A. (1988) Health. In *Britain's Black Population: A New Perspective* (eds A. Bhat, P. Carrhill and S. Ohri), (2nd edn), Radical Statistics Race Group, Gower, Aldershot

Gunaratnam, Y. (1993) Breaking the silence: Asian carers in Britain. In *Community Care*, (eds J. Bornat, C. Pereira, D. Pilgrim and F. Williams), Macmillan, London

Hill, M. (1990) Independent Living for black and ethnic minority disabled people. In *Building Our Lives*, (ed. L. Laurie), Shelter, London

Hill, M. (1991) Race and disability. In the book of readings of the disability equality pack *Disability—Identity, Sexuality and Relationships* K665y, Open University, Milton Keynes

Holden, G. (1988) Why are people from ethnic minorities losing out? *Disability Now*, August, 8–9

Hugman, R. (1991) *Power in Caring Professions*, Macmillan, London

Javed, K. (1993) *Survey into the Needs of Visually Impaired Asians*, Association of Blind Asians, London

Jeewa, M. (1990) Asian people with disabilities alliance. In *Building Our Lives*, (ed. L. Laurie), Shelter, London

Kroll, D. (1990) Equal access to care. *Nursing Times*, **86 (23)**, 72–73

Ley, P. (1988) *Communicating with Patients*, Croom Helm, London

London Borough's Disability Resource Team (1991) *Disability Equality Training Trainers' Guide*, Central Council for Education and Training in Social Work, London

Lonsdale, S. (1990) *Women and Disability*, Macmillan, London

McCalman, J. A. (1990) *The Forgotten People*, King's Fund Centre/Help the Aged/Standing Conference for Ethnic Minority Senior Citizens, London

McDonald, P. (1991) Double discrimination must be faced now. *Disability Now*, 8 March

McGee, P. (1992) *Teaching Transcultural Care*, Chapman & Hall, London

Melzeck, R. and Wall, P. (1988) *The Challenge of Pain*, Penguin Books, Harmondsworth

Mosaic (1991) BBC1, 24 February

Oliver, M. (1990) *The Politics of Disablement*, Macmillan, London

Open University (1990) *Disability—Changing Practice*, Disability Equality Training Pack, (K665x) Open University, Milton Keynes

Patel, K (1992) On the margins: ethnic minority groups and services for visual impairment. *The New Beacon*, **76 (896)**, 90–93

Rack, P. (1982) *Race, Culture and Mental Disorder*, Tavistock, London

RADAR (undated) *Ethnic Minority Groups and People with Disabilities*, Royal Association for Disability and Rehabilitation, London

Read, J. (1988) *The Equal Opportunities Book*, InterChange Books, London

Sickle Cell Society (1990), London, personal communication

Simes, L. (1990) Partnership with parents—a positive example. In *Asian Children and Special Needs: A Report for ACE*, (ed. C. Orton), Advisory Centre for Education, London

Smith, A. and Jacobson, B. (1988) *The Nation's Health*, King's Fund Publishing Office, London

Stokes, J. (1988) Breaking the ethnic language barrier. *Therapy Weekly*, **14 (31)**, 7

Stuart, O. (1993) Double oppression: an appropriate starting point? In *Disabling Barriers—Enabling Environments*, (eds J. Swain, V. Finkelstein, S. French and M. Oliver), Sage, London

Therapy Weekly (1991) Deaf Minorities ned speach therapy, **17 (35)**, 20

Tomlinson, S. (1990) Asian children with special needs—A Broad perspective. In *Asian Children and Special Needs: A Report for ACE*, (ed. C. Orton), Advisory Centre for Education, London

Vousden, M. (1987) Racism in the wards. *Nursing Times*, **83 (42)**, 918

Watkins, S. (1987) *Medicine and Labour*, Lawrence Wishart, London

Weller, B. (1991) Nursing in a multicultural world. *Nursing Standard*, **5 (30)**, 31–32

Whitehead, M. (1988) *Inequalities in Health: The Health Divide*, Penguin Books, Harmondsworth

Wilson, L. (1989) Dilemma of 172 recorded languages. *Therapy Weekly*, **16 (20)**, 3

Many of the ideas in this chapter are based upon meetings, which took place in 1990 and 1991, with the following organizations:

Association of Blind Asians
Sickle Cell Society
Asian People with Disabilities Alliance
Jewish Blind Society
Association for the Support of Asian Parents of Handicapped People

Thanks are extended to these organizations for their time and assistance.

14

Abuse of children and adults who are disabled

Helen Westcott

This chapter discusses the abuse of disabled children and adults. Its primary focus is on the forms of child abuse labelled 'physical, sexual, emotional abuse and neglect'. However, the rights of disabled people are abused in their everyday lives (they are discriminated against) and this contributes to the societal context within which child abuse occurs. In this chapter I have drawn on my own research (Westcott, 1993) concerning the abuse of children and adults who are disabled, as well as 'borrowing' heavily from a number of professionals who have experience of this issue (eg Kennedy, 1989; Marchant and Page, 1993). It should be noted at the outset that this chapter will not address issues specific to the abuse of disabled children who are black or from minority ethnic groups, although much will be relevant to them as children who are disabled. Much greater understanding of their particular needs, and experiences of multiple oppression, is required (see also chapter 13 of this book.)

Vulnerability of disabled children and adults

Fundamentally, society creates the vulnerability of disabled people through the maintenance of stereotypes, prejudices and discrimination against people who are disabled. The use of the term 'vulnerability' may be problematic, since the concept takes the existence of abuse for granted, and focuses on the question of 'why these victims?' rather than 'why abuse?' (Kelly, May 1993, personal communication). Thus attention must be paid to how abusers (especially sexual abusers) can target certain children and adults (eg those who are disabled), and to how opportunities for abuse are created. Unfortunately, and especially within institutional and medical settings, there are many examples of how this can occur.

Isolation and segregation

Disabled people are, on the whole, rejected by society, and frequently are segregated in 'special' homes, schools and institutions (Ammerman, Lubetsky and Drudy, 1991). Use of residential care by itself appears to increase the opportunities for abuse, as illustrated in recent 'scandals' such as 'Pindown' (Levy and Kahan, 1991). Some cases have involved people who have impairments (eg Scotforth House, Lancaster, and Lordship Lane Hostel, Southwark).[1]

The isolation frequently enforced upon residents of homes, boarding schools, etc makes it difficult to establish links with the local community, and to identify people outside the institution who may be able to help (see Westcott, 1991b, for a review). It also undermines their self-esteem and lowers their quality of life through restricted access to social and recreational facilities (Solomons, Abel and Epley, 1981). Children and young people in institutional care can be rendered extremely powerless; this coupled with their isolation makes them easy victims for those wishing to abuse them. This was recently highlighted by another residential care scandal, in Leicestershire, involving the abusive regime perpetrated by Frank Beck (Kirkwood, 1993).

Exclusion from mainstream services and facilities

There are many examples of the ways in which disabled children and adults remain excluded from mainstream services, eg through the inaccessibility of education and housing. Where disabled children are educated at special schools, further opportunities for abuse are created by the unsupervised transport of children in buses and taxis to the schools, and the lack of vetting of drivers (Cohen and Warren, 1990).

Child protection services are generally poorly equipped to handle referrals concerning children who are disabled: there may even be professional denial that disabled children are at risk of abuse in the first place (Marchant, 1991). As well as being physically inaccessible (video interviewing suites inevitably seem destined for the first floor, without lifts or loop systems[2]), services are typically communicatively inaccessible. Child protection social workers have little training or knowledge about working with disabled children, and a 'gap' in knowledge and skills exists between the worlds of child protection and child disability (Marchant and Page, 1993). It is not surprising, then, when disabled children fall through this gap, and fail to be identified as at risk by professionals from any agency. Young people who are disabled are particularly vulnerable in this respect (Russell, 1991; Westcott, 1993).

Experiences with medical professionals

As a result of their physical impairment(s), children and adults who are disabled will experience much greater contact with a range of different medical professionals, including nurses, doctors, occupational therapists, speech therapists and physiotherapists. Harrison (1993) discusses the medical philosophy and culture which has dictated the generally patronizing and insensitive way in which disabled people are responded to. Disabled people frequently experience their contacts with medical professionals as intrusive and abusive (eg Cross, 1990), and more opportunities for physical, sexual and emotional abuse and neglect of children are created.

In my own research, thirty-four adults who had been abused as children were interviewed (Westcott, 1993). Of these, seventeen interviewees had a physical or learning impairment; the perpetrators included a hospital porter (n=1), physiotherapists (n=3), and other hospital staff (n=9), These interviewees had been subjected to all forms of child abuse, and for some their abuse had continued into adulthood.

Experiences with health organizations had been traumatic for many of the people I spoke to, especially where the perpetrators were themselves associated with the profession. Some comments from the victims themselves may help to illustrate:

> If I was at all noisy they would take my bed—they would put it into the garden store at the end of the ward and it wasn't even a proper room, it was brickwork . . . it was dark, it was bricks, there were tools all around, they used to literally wheel me in there and lock me in and the gardener hated it . . . it was terrifying.
> (Woman with cerebral palsy abused by hospital staff)

> I was put in straitjacket. I just cracked up in side room. Trying to get ways to tell people what was happening. Punishment was to scrub floors with scrubbing brush. They kept hitting me across face with towels, stripped me of my clothes—had to wear pyjamas.
> (Man with learning difficulties abused by hospital staff)

> It started when I was sixteen years old. They took advantage of me and so I'm not a virgin anymore. They were supposed to do exercises with me and they did other things instead.
> (Woman with cerebral palsy abused by physiotherapists) (Westcott, 1993; 16–17)

The way in which general medical experiences can lead to disabled people being made vulnerable to abusive acts was graphically illustrated by the comments of a woman who had polio as a child. She was sexually abused by a porter during one of her many stays in hospital.

The medical experiences I had made me very vulnerable to being abused it just seemed the same as everything else that had been done to me, so I wasn't able to discriminate . . . there's no way you can say no to what a doctor does to you they just damn well do it when you're a kid you don't have any choice about it. . . . What the doctors did, they lifted up my nightdress, they poked her and they pushed her without asking me, without doing anything, but in front of a load of other people it was absolutely no different, I didn't say no to any doctor, the porter actually was to me doing absolutely nothing different at all that every doctor or nurses had ever done. (Westcott, 1993: 17)

Care is needed in interpreting this quote; it does not suggest that disabled people are unable to recognize when they are being abused—as the previous quotations illustrate. It does, however, highlight the lack of choice disabled children experience over what is happening to them, and the profound and negative effects frequent hospitalizations can have.

Provision of intimate care

Many disabled children and adults require assistance with intimate care activities such as washing, dressing and using the toilet. All these activities create opportunities for the disabled person to be abused—care may be appropriately provided on a one-to-one basis in a private room, but a child is often not given a choice about who performs the tasks. Several children and young people subject to the investigations carried out by Marchant and Page (1992; 1993) had been abused during intimate care activities, whether in their home or in residential care.

The above discussions highlight some of the ways in which opportunities for the abuse of disabled children and adults are created. There are other factors which contribute: poor vetting of residential care staff which enables paedophiles and abusers to obtain employment (Westcott, 1991b); poor quality general and sexual education experienced by disabled people; failure to provide children and adults who use alternative communication systems with a necessary vocabulary to describe abuse (Kennedy, 1992; Marchant and Page, 1992; 1993). Underlying all these issues is the fundamental powerlessness of children, and of disabled people, as a result of their oppression by a predominantly adult, 'able-bodied' society.

Prevalence estimates for abuse of disabled children

A number of studies have investigated the abuse of children who are disabled (see Ammerman, Van Hasselt and Hersen, 1988; Kelly, 1992;

Westcott, 1991a; White, Benedict, Wulff and Kelley, 1987 for reviews). Many of these studies have a number of methodological shortcomings which need to be considered (see Kelly, 1992; Westcott, 1991a). Not least among these is the failure to involve disabled people themselves in the research (see chapter 10). There are no research data currently available which conclusively prove that disabled children are abused more than non-disabled children, although there is now a considerable number of studies which suggest this is the case. The lack of any prevalence studies or national incidence data[3] relating to this issue is a major research gap; the government's own figures regarding children on child protection registers do not contain data on whether or not the child has an impairment.

Most prevalence studies to date have looked at abuse retrospectively in selected groups of disabled young people or adults. Other studies have examined groups of abused children to see how many were disabled before and/or after the abuse. Definitions of abuse and disability have varied across studies so that generalizations must be tentative. In addition, the majority of research to date has been conducted in America, although some British studies are available.

In 1977, Buchanan and Oliver looked at the medical and social records and clinical assessments of 140 children who had learning difficulties and were aged under 16 years in an English hospital. Twenty-two per cent of the children were victims of physical abuse, with a further 10 per cent judged 'at risk'. For 3 per cent of the children definitely—and 11 per cent probably—their abuse had caused their impairment. Glaser and Bentovim (1979) studied the records of 174 children aged up to 10 years in a London hospital. The children were 'moderately to severely' physically or learning disabled, or chronically sick. Forty-six per cent of the disabled or sick children had been physically abused (29 per cent) or neglected (71 per cent). Kennedy (1989) surveyed 156 teachers and social workers with deaf people in the United Kingdom. These respondents knew of 136 deaf children who had been 'confirmed' abused, and a further 262 deaf children were suspected victims. This included physical, sexual and emotional abuse.

Newport (1991) studied 57 disabled children who had received day care from a Barnardo's project. Of these, 35 children (61 per cent) could be described as having been abused, according to Newport's definition. The abusive acts included physical and emotional abuse, neglect, lack of stimulation, over protection, confinement (to room/cot), lack of supervision, drugs given incorrectly and insufficient treatment (see Newport, 1991: 7). The most frequent type of abuse suffered was 'lack of stimulation' (n=12, 34 per cent). Newport's helpful expansion of her definition of abuse is especially relevant for disabled children; acts such as 'lack of stimulation', 'over protection' and 'drugs given incorrectly' may be particularly important, and not applicable to non-disabled children. My own research suggests that definitions of physical abuse may need to be revised for disabled people—for example, to include their experiences of normalization.[4] Such definitions would embrace 'inappropriate, especially pain inducing treatment to achieve "normality" ' for instance (Westcott, 1993).

The above studies have been cited as examples of British research with different children, different research methods and different rates of abuse. As previously noted, more comprehensive reviews are available elsewhere (Ammerman et al., 1988; Kelly, 1992; Westcott, 1991a; White et al., 1987). In her review Kelly (1992) reports prevalence estimates of 25 to 83 per cent for the abuse of children who are disabled, and my own review (in 1991a) gave estimates ranging from 10.6 per cent to 83 per cent.[5] Clearly, disabled children are being abused, and the issue demands proper prevalence and incidence figures.

Effects of abuse

Disabled victims of abuse have reported similar short and long-term effects of child abuse as their non-disabled peers (Westcott, 1993). Some authors have further argued that the effects of sexual abuse may be more severe for adults who have learning difficulties (eg Tharinger, Horton and Millea, 1990). Physical after effects can include sickness and ill health, weight problems and psychosomatic disorders. Psychologically, the victim may have great difficulties in forming stable relationships, and in enabling trust to develop (see Hevey and Kenward, 1992; Kenward and Hevey, 1992, for reviews).

Finkelhor and Browne (1985) discuss four traumagenics of child sexual abuse which give rise to the harmful effects: traumatic sexualization, betrayal, powerlessness and stigmatization. Traumatic sexualization refers to a process whereby a child's sexuality is shaped in a developmentally inappropriate manner as a result of sexual abuse. Betrayal occurs where children discover that someone on whom they were 'vitally dependent' has caused them harm. Powerlessness refers to a process in which a child's will and decisions are continually infringed. Finally, stigmatization refers to the negative feelings (badness, shame and guilt) communicated to the child that give rise to poor self-esteem and social isolation.

Finkelhor and Browne (1985) argue that these individual traumagenics are not unique to sexual abuse, but their 'conjunction' in one set of circumstances (ie sexual abuse) is. In my research, all disabled and non-disabled interviewees reported at least one of the traumagenics to some degree, irrespective of abuse experienced (Westcott, 1993). Interviewees who were disabled especially described feelings of vulnerability, and interviewees with learning difficulties seemed extremely powerless (both in their own perceptions and in their actual circumstances). Even during the research interview, many years after they had been abused, they still demonstrated a strong fear of repercussions for telling about what had happened:

> Frightened to tell social worker in case it got back to the home. Threats— I'll go back to the hospital, I'll leave home. Get me somewhere to live where I won't get picked on when don't take tablets.

> Dare not tell because everybody had some drugs. Told doctor I didn't have any marks but when I went to hospital I had. I was too scared to tell them.
> (Two men with learning difficulties, physically assaulted by care staff; Westcott, 1993: 22)

The interaction between abuse, disability and occupation was illustrated by the position of one male disabled interviewee. As a result of the assault perpetrated upon him, his impairment (epilepsy) was exacerbated resulting in the repeated loss of employment (through prejudicial reactions of employers). Clearly there may be consequences for disabled people who are abused which arise as a result of both the specific abusive act (eg rape, physical assault) perpetrated upon them, and also from their general life experiences of being disabled (eg oppression, discrimination).

Recognizing and responding to possible child abuse

Signs of possible abuse

A recent book has highlighted key issues in child protection for nurses and health visitors (Naish and Cloke, 1992), and several introductory reviews are available which discuss the recognition of child abuse in its different forms (eg Bannister, 1992; Stern, 1987). Table 1 presents some of the more obvious physical and behavioural signs which may indicate a child is being abused. However, this is *not* a definitive guide, and a range of factors should be considered: for example, the child's age, personal history, family circumstances, current situation. It is also important to consider whether such signs could result from the child's experience of being disabled (see below).

The signs and indicators presented in Table 14.1 may be more or less specific to different types of abuse. Physical abuse or neglect is likely to result in physical injuries such as bruises or fractures, but physical injuries can also result from sexual abuse, eg bruising to

Table 14.1 Signs of Possible Child Abuse

Physical Signs	Behavioural Signs
Hand-slap marks	Pseudomature, sexually explicit
Bruising of mouth or cheeks	behaviour
Grip marks on arms or trunk	Continual open masturbation or
Black eyes	aggressive sex play with peers
Bruising to breasts, buttocks,	Overly compliant or 'watchful attitude'
thighs, genital or rectal areas	Acting out aggressive behaviour
Burns and scalds	Air of detachment
Fractures	Isolation
Bite marks	Not trusting anyone
Poisoning	Psychosomatic pains
Sexually transmitted disease	Eating disorders
	Sleeping disturbance, bedwetting or
	nightmares
	Clinical depression
	Disclosure by child

Table derived from Bannister (1992)

genital or rectal areas, or presence of a sexually transmitted disease (STD). Similarly, behavioural indicators are more usually associated with sexual abuse, eg overly compliant behaviour or aggressive acting out, but these same signs could result from a child being physically mistreated. Again, care is needed to consider all the issues, including the possibility that the injury was accidentally caused, or that a different stressor (eg parental separation, a death in the family, or another significant life event) has led to the child's behaviour changing.

Abuse and disability as causes of a child's behaviour

Where the child has an impairment, recognizing child abuse is considerably more complicated. One reason for this is a need for a more specialized assessment of possible indicators, especially if the child has multiple impairments (Marchant and Page, 1993)—the professional involved must disentangle the dual aetiology of the child's behavioural or emotional responses (Kennedy, 1990).

Kennedy (1990) has discussed how a deaf child may experience similar emotions as a result of being abused or of being deaf. Her arguments can be applied to any child who is disabled and relate to different forms of abuse. Thus possible experiences for the child, including isolation, rejection and confusion may stem from both the oppression of disabled people and/or from the abusive act. Kennedy lists many examples of this dual aetiology, including the following:

Self-blame: 'I've caused all the family problems by being deaf.'
             'I've caused all the problems by being abused.'
Frustration: 'I can't hear.' 'I don't understand.'
             'How do I stop it?' 'How do I get away?'
Confusion: 'What's happening?' 'Why am I deaf?'
             'What's happening?' 'Why is this happening?'
(Kennedy, 1990: 5)

In their investigations of suspected abuse among children with multiple impairments, Marchant and Page (1993) considered a number of factors in assessing the level of concern about a particular child, and in assessing the need to investigate further. The four categories of concerns were a disclosure or allegation by a child to another person; emotional, behavioural or medical signs or symptoms; contact with a known or suspected abuser; abuse being witnessed and reported by a third party.

The first two categories have already been discussed, and apply to disabled children as for non-disabled children. It is worth stressing, however, the particular difficulties facing some disabled children who may wish to make a disclosure: specifically, those using augmentative communication systems.[6] Many such systems do not have the necessary vocabulary to describe either private body parts or abusive acts. It is also notable that those adults best placed to notice changes in a child's emotional, behavioural or physical well being will include professionals not necessarily in contact with social workers or child protection professionals—eg speech therapists, occupational therapists, teachers, paediatricians, etc.

Marchant and Page's (1993) third category for assessing suspicion was known contact with a suspected abuser. Although they acknowledge that using this criterion can be viewed as problematic, they stress its importance for disabled children; it was the only grounds for suspecting abuse with nine of the fifteen children involved in their investigations, but it was found to be a very significant predictor of risk. Where a suspected abuser had contact with a large number of children, a risk continuum was developed to estimate the risk for individual children. This ranged from 'high risk: regular unsupervised contact including intimate care' to the 'no risk: no unsupervised contact or no contact at all' (see Marchant and Page, 1993: 9–10, for full details).

The final category was that of 'abuse witnessed and reported by a third party'—information from a child who witnesses abuse of another child. Marchant and Page argue this may be particularly relevant for disabled children using residential or respite care for a number of reasons: the lack of privacy and shared facilities; increased sense of responsibility for others as a result of living together; recognition by the children of their different abilities to communicate.

Taken together, then, these categories could lead to a 'high index of concern' that a child was being abused.

Professionals working with abused and/or disabled children must develop the awareness that disability and abuse are not exclusive, and that when assessing a child's behaviour and responses both possibilities need to be borne in mind. To this end, the Department of Health has funded the development of a training pack 'ABuse and Children who are Disabled (ABCD)'— published in November 1993. This pack provides relevant material for professionals from both child protection and child disability backgrounds. (Useful addresses for relevant agencies are also provided in the Appendix).

Responding to possible abuse

In many ways, nurses and therapists in regular contact with children are ideally placed to notice any unusual physical or social signs (such as changes in a child's behaviour) that may indicate a child is being abused or is at risk. For example, midwives and health visitors can encourage parents to seek help and support when they are experiencing difficulties, and so prevent abuse. Nurses in hospitals can be alert to parents who 'shop around for medical services to conceal the repeated nature of their child's injuries' (Department of Health, 1991; 18). School nurses can monitor children's health and development. Any suspicions should be discussed with a senior colleague, and passed on to an appropriate statutory authority (Social Services Department, Police or NSPCC). Investigating allegations of child abuse is a skilled undertaking, and the nurse or therapist should not take it upon themselves to perform the role of investigator.

If a child discloses abuse, or indicates that he/she wishes to talk, the nurse or therapist should:

- listen to the child, rather than directly question him or her;
- never stop a child who is freely recalling significant events;
- make a note of the discussion, taking care to record the timing, setting and personnel present as well as what was said.
  (Home Office, 1992; 6)

It is important to remember the following:

- take what the child says seriously;
- react calmly;
- tell the child that he or she is not to blame;
- explain to the child what will happen next;

- check out your understanding with the child of what has happened, if you are unclear about what the child is saying;
- keep questions to a minimum;
- never ask leading questions or make assumptions;
- use the words the child uses (eg for different parts of the body). (see NSPCC, 1989: 9–12)

Local procedures and guidance for investigating allegations of abuse are issued by the relevant Area Child Protection Committee (ACPC), and these in turn will be based upon governmental guidance issued in *Working Together* (Department of Health, 1991). *Working Together* states that 'interdisciplinary and interagency work is an essential process in the task of attempting to protect children from abuse' (Department of Health, 1991: 5). Area Child Protection Committees (ACPCs) provide a 'joint forum for developing, monitoring and reviewing child protection policies', and are made up of representatives from social services, police, health and education.

Working Together spells out the roles and responsibilities of the health services, including the district health authority, midwife and health visitor, hospital staff, primary and community health services, child and adolescent mental health service, family health service authorities, general practitioners and private health care. Further guidance has been issued specifically for senior nurses, health visitors and midwives (Department of Health, 1992). All nurses and therapists should be familiar with the relevant sections of these documents, and in addition should refer to their own professional guidelines regarding abuse (see, for example, The College of Speech and Language Therapists, 1991).

Improving practice

There are several ways in which nurses and therapists can start to think about improving their practice. These include developing their knowledge of disability and their awareness of their own attitudes and prejudices towards disabled people, as well as promoting anti-discriminatory practice by everyone concerned. However, the most effective way to improve practice will be to listen to the experiences of disabled children and adults themselves, and to amend and improve services accordingly. Professionals should also sensitize themselves to the possibility that, like all children, disabled children may be abused by those who care for them, be it parents, carers or professional colleagues.

Silburn (1993) describes how therapy services for disabled people in Derbyshire were overhauled to make them community based, appropriate and accessible to those disabled people who required them. Cross (1992) has provided guidelines for the provision of sensitive medical examinations and treatment. The Child Protection Working Group at Chailey Heritage Children's Centre has also produced 'Guidelines and Policies Relating to Child Protection' (1992). They include guidelines for good practice in the provision of intimate care. These are just a few examples of how practice can be improved; obviously, much more is required, and it is the responsibility of *all* professionals to ensure that it is achieved.

Conclusion

This chapter has reviewed a number of issues relating to the abuse of children and adults who are disabled. Prevalence studies have indicated that many disabled children are abused, and action is needed now to prevent this from continuing. A failure to understand the issues discussed here continues to place disabled children at risk of abuse. Professionals must consider the way in which society creates both disability and vulnerability.

Disabled people should not be isolated or segregated from the community in which they live, and disablist and racist practice in service provision must be stopped.[7] Medical organizations and professionals need to assess and improve the way in which they respond to disabled children and adults, and carers should recognize the difficulties inherent in providing intimate care. Other practical steps include better vetting of professionals responsible for the care of disabled children, and the provision of an adequate vocabulary for people using alternative systems of communication.

Nurses and therapists are well placed to recognize possible indicators of abuse, but identification is considerably more complicated when the child has an impairment. Professionals working in child protection and with children who are disabled need to recognize the risks to disabled children, and work together to protect them from abuse. Abuse must be considered in the context of the child's life experiences, including their impairment, race, culture and gender.

Individual practitioners are responsible for improving their own practice, and managers for implementing anti-discriminatory policies and services. An understanding of the societal context in which disabled people are abused is fundamental to the development of such services, and to the safeguarding of disabled children's welfare.

Notes

[1] For reports see *The Guardian*, 24 November 1992 'Incompetent Council let children suffer' and *The Times*, 24 February 1993, 'Staff at Council home sacked for abusing mentally handicapped'.

[2] For partially deaf children and young people.

[3] Incidence studies of child abuse count the number of new cases of child abuse in any one year. Prevalence studies of child abuse examine the proportion of the general population who have experienced abuse.

[4] I am using the term normalization here to refer to the process whereby attempts are made to eradicate the person's impairment or to 'overcome' it. For example, repeated operations on 'club feet' in an attempt to make the child walk as a 'normal' non-disabled child.

[5] Recent work in Britain investigating *sexual* abuse amongst *adults* who have a learning disability found 23 per cent of their sample had experienced non-contact sexual abuse, and 95 per cent had experienced contact sexual abuse (Brown and Turk, 1992; Turk and Brown, 1992).

[6] For example, Bliss, Makaton or Rebus. See Kennedy (1992).

[7] There are possible exceptions, where it is to the advantage of certain groups to receive dedicated services. For example, the education of deaf children.

References

Ammerman, R. T., Lubetsky, M. J. and Drudy, K. F. (1991) Maltreatment of handicapped children. In *Case Studies in Family Violence*, (eds R. T. Ammerman and M. Hersen), Plenum Press, New York

Ammerman, R. T., Van Hasselt, V. B. and Hersen, M. (1988) Maltreatment of handicapped children: a critical review. *Journal of Family Violence*, **3 (1)**, 53–72

Bannister, A. (1992) Recognising abuse. In *Child Abuse and Neglect: Facing the Challenge*, (eds W. Stainton Rogers, D. Hevey, J. Roche and E. Ash), B. T. Batsford Ltd, London

Brown, H. and Turk, V. (1992) Defining sexual abuse as it affects adults with learning disabilities. *Mental Handicap*, **20**, 44–55

Buchanan, A. and Oliver, J. E. (1977) Abuse and neglect as cause of mental retardation: a study of 140 children admitted to subnormality hospitals in Wiltshire. *British Journal of Psychiatry*, **131**, 458–467

Chailey Heritage Child Protection Working Group (1992) *Guidelines and Policies Relating to Child Protection*, Chailey Heritage, North Chailey, East Sussex

Cohen, S. and Warren, R. D. (1990) The intersection of disability and child abuse in England and the United States. *Child Welfare*, **69**, 253–262

The College of Speech and Language Therapists (1991) *Communicating Quality: Professional Standards for Speech and Language Therapists*, The College of Speech and Language Therapists, London

Cross, M. (1990) Perspectives of disability. In *Abused Children with Disabilities: Notes of the Seminar*, London Borough of Croydon, London

Cross, M. (1992) Abusive practices and disempowerment of children with physical impairments. *Child Abuse Review*, **1 (3)**, 194–197

Department of Health (1991) *Working Together Under the Children Act 1989: A Guide for Inter-Agency Co-operation for the Protection of Children from Abuse*, HMSO, London

Department of Health (1992) *Child Protection: Guidance for Senior Nurses, Health Visitors and Midwives*, HMSO, London

Finkelhor, D. and Browne, A. (1985) The traumatic impact of child sexual abuse: a conceptualization. *American Journal of Orthopsychiatry*, **55**, 530–541

Glaser, D. and Bentovim, A. (1979) Abuse and risk to handicapped and chronically ill children. *Child Abuse and Neglect*, **3**, 565–575

Harrison, J. (1993) Medical responsibilities to disabled people. In *Disabling Barriers—Enabling Environments*, (eds J. Swain, V. Finkelstein, S. French and M. Oliver), Sage, London

Hevey, D. and Kenward, H. (1992) The effects of child sexual abuse. In *Child Abuse and Neglect: Facing the Challenge*, (eds W. Stainton Rogers, D. Hevey, J. Roche and E. Ash), B. T. Batsford Ltd, London

Home Office in conjunction with Department of Health (1992) *Memorandum of Good Practice on Video Recorded Interviews with Child Witnesses for Criminal Proceedings*, HMSO, London

Kelly, L. (1992) The connections between disability and child abuse: a review of the research evidence. *Child Abuse Review*, **1 (3)**, 157–169

Kennedy, M. (1989) The abuse of deaf children. *Child Abuse Review*, **3 (1)**, 3–7

Kennedy, M. (1990) The deaf child who is sexually abused—is there a need for a dual specialist? *Child Abuse Review*, **4 (2)**, 3–6

Kennedy, M. (1992) Not the only way to communicate: a challenge to voice in child protection work. *Child Abuse Review*, **1 (3)**, 169–178

Kenward, H. and Hevey, D. (1992) The effects of physical abuse and neglect. In *Child Abuse and Neglect: Facing the Challenge*, (eds W. Stainton Rogers, D. Hevey, J. Roche and E. Ash), B. T. Batsford Ltd, London

Kirkwood, A. (1993) *The Leicestershire Inquiry 1992*, Leicestershire County Council, Leicester

Levy, A. and Kahan, B. (1991) *The Pindown Experience and the Protection of Children: The Report of the Staffordshire Child Care Inquiry*, Staffordshire County Council, Stafford

Marchant, R. (1991) Myths and facts about sexual abuse and children with disabilities. *Child Abuse Review*, **5 (2)**, 22–24

Marchant, R. and Page, M. (1992) Bridging the gap: investigating the abuse of children with multiple disabilities. *Child Abuse Review*, **1 (3)**, 179–183

Marchant, R. and Page, M. (1993) *Bridging the Gap: Child protection Work with Children with Multiple Disabilities*, NSPCC, London

Naish, J. and Cloke, C. (1992) *Key Issues in Child Protection for Health Visitors and Nurses*, Longman, Harlow

National Society for the Prevention of Cruelty to Children (1989) *Protecting Children: A Guide for Teachers on Child Abuse*, NSPCC, London

Newport, P. (1991) *Linking Child Abuse With Disability*, Barnardos, London

Russell, P. (1991) Working with children with physical disabilities and their families—the social work role. In *Social Work: Disabled People and Disabling Environments*, (ed. M. Oliver), Jessica Kingsley, London

Silburn, L. (1993) A social model in a medical world: the development of the integrated living team as part of the strategy for younger physically disabled people in North Derbyshire. In *Disabling Barriers—Enabling Environments*, (eds J. Swain, V. Finkelstein, S. French and M. Oliver), Sage, London

Solomons, G., Abel, C. M. and Epley, S. (1981) A community development approach to the prevention of institutional and societal child maltreatment. *Child Abuse and Neglect*, **5**, 135–140

Stern, C. (1987) The recognition of child abuse. In *Child Abuse: The Educational Perspective*, (ed. P. Maher), Blackwell, Oxford

Tharinger, D., Horton, C. B. and Millea, S. (1990) Sexual abuse and exploitation of children and adults with mental retardation and other handicaps. *Child Abuse and Neglect*, **14**, 301–312

Turk, V. and Brown, H. (1992) Sexual abuse and adults with learning disabilities: preliminary communication of survey results. *Mental Handicap*, **20**, 55–58

Westcott, H. L. (1991a) The abuse of disabled children: a review of the literature. *Child: Care, Health and Development*, **17 (4)**, 243–258

Westcott, H. L. (1991b) *Institutional Abuse of Children—From Research to Policy: A Review*, NSPCC, London

Westcott, H. L. (1993) *Abuse of Children and Adults with Disabilities*, NSPCC, London

White, R. B., Benedict, M. I., Wulff, L. M. and Kelley, M. (1987) Physical disabilities as risk factors for child maltreatment: a selected review. *Child Abuse and Neglect*, **5**, 135–140

Acknowledgements

I would like to thank Kevin Barrett and Marcus Page for their helpful and constructive comments on earlier drafts of this chapter.

Appendix: organizations working with abused disabled children and adults

National Association for the Protection from Sexual Abuse of Adults and Children with Learning Difficulties (NAPSAC)
Development Officer: Pam Cooke
Department of Mental Handicap
University of Nottingham Medical School
Queens Medical Centre
Nottingham
NG7 2UH

Telephone: 0602 421421 extension 44524

National Deaf Children's Society
Keep Deaf Children Safe Project (KDCS)
Co-ordinator: Margaret Kennedy
Nuffield Hearing and Speech Centre
325 Gray's Inn Road
London
WC1X 0DA

Telephone: 071 833 5627

RESPOND
Steve Morris and Tamsin Cottis
170 Garratt Lane
Wandsworth
London
SW18

Telephone: 081 877 9992/081 870 7171

15

Gender and disability

Jenny Morris

Introduction

When thinking about gender and disability it is important to be clear what we mean by these terms. The tendency to confuse sex and gender is similar to the tendency to confuse impairment and disability. Both sex and impairment are characteristics relating to the human body, the one concerning reproductive functions, the other concerning functional limitations (physical, sensory or intellectual). On the other hand, both gender and disability are social constructs. Gender concerns what it is to be male or female in a particular social context while disability concerns the way that a society reacts to impairment. The concept of gender explains the different social, economic and political experiences of men and women; the concept of disability explains the social, economic and political experiences associated with impairment.

In each case, there is an interaction between physical characteristics and the social context in which they occur. For example, childbirth is a physical experience which can be life-threatening. The nature of the experience and the extent to which it is life-threatening will vary according to factors such as the woman's material well-being and the health services available. Limb amputation is similarly a physical experience which may be life-threatening, but the nature of the experience is to a large extent determined by the social context in which it takes place; we only have to consider the situation of someone having a limb amputated in Bosnia in 1993 to recognize the importance of social context.

However, gender and disability as social constructs particularly come into play when we consider the *consequences* of physical events such as childbirth or limb amputation. The physical act of giving birth does not in itself determine either the nature of the relationship between mother and child or the effect on the mother's lifestyle or life chances. These will be determined by many different factors such as the general social status of mothers, the material consequences of having a child, the involvement of men in parenting, the availability of help with child care, employment opportunities for women with children. Similarly, the experience of limb amputation does not in itself determine what lacking an arm or a leg means to the individual concerned nor its effect on his or her lifestyle or life chances. These things will vary according to factors such as what resources society puts into mobility equipment, employers' attitudes towards mobility impairment, whether social attitudes mean that limb deficiency provokes ridicule, pity or hostility.

Both gender and disability have been developed as tools for analysing and explaining an experience of inequality. The sexual division of child care and the consequences for women are thus explained, not in terms of women's biological role in reproduction but in terms of the way societies organize child care. In western societies, these arrangements are seen to result in an experience of economic inequality—in comparison with men—which has a number of consequences for women's health, social status and life chances generally.

Disability is a conceptual tool developed by the disabled people's movement to explain an experience of inequality which people with impairments experience in comparison with those who do not have impairments. For example, western society's reliance on the printed word for communication does not disable those who can see to read but it does disable—in the sense that it marginalizes, excludes—those who cannot see to read the printed word. Thus it is disability which determines the social and economic consequences of visual impairment rather than the impairment itself.

There is very little written about the relationship between gender and disability, and that which there is tends to focus on the experience of disabled women, presenting them as 'suffering from a double handicap' (see, for example, Hanna and Rogovsky, 1991). This chapter attempts to resist this rather simplistic categorization, partly because such an approach is bound to obscure the relationship between gender and disability in men's experience, but also because this way of describing disabled women turns them into passive victims of insurmountable oppression.

The chapter is concerned with looking at the relationship between gender and disability from two angles: firstly, the ways in which sex and gender influence the experience of impairment and disability; and secondly, the ways in which impairment and disability influence the experience of being male or female.

The influence of sex and gender on impairment and disability

Sex, gender and the incidence of impairment

Sex and gender influence both the prevalence of impairment and its causes. The most recent large-scale survey of people with impairments in Britain found that there were 3,656,000 women who experienced restrictions in their daily lives as a result of impairment compared with 2,544,000 men (OPCS, 1988a). The risk of impairment increases with age and this numerical difference is therefore partly accounted for by the fact that on average women live longer than men. However, prevalence rates of impairment are also higher among women than amongst men in the 16 to 59 age group.

There are also differences in the causes of impairment among men and women, with women being more likely to experience 'locomotor conditions, mainly arthritic diseases, and more conditions associated with dementia. Men report significantly more respiratory conditions and more injuries' (Patrick, 1989: 29). These differences in the causes of impairment among men and women would appear to account at least partly for the higher level of impairment among women, for there is evidence that men are more likely to experience conditions which lead to early death, whereas women are more likely to experience conditions which are not life threatening but result in many years of living with impairment (Arber and Ginn, 1991: 113).

Some of the differences in the incidence and cause of impairment among men and women are biological in origin—breast cancer and haemophilia, for example. And certain aspects of the differences in incidence and cause of impairment are determined by a combination of biological and social factors. For instance, the greater longevity among women is partly biologically determined (as discussed by Hart, 1989) and partly created by men's higher risk of dying at earlier ages through occupational diseases and accidents (these features being a consequence of men's role in our society).

A major contribution to the higher incidence of impairment among women must, however, be the way that gender inequalities influence women's health. It has been argued that women are generally at a greater risk of ill health because of the way that gender inequalities result in a higher risk of poverty for women. Factors such as women's position within the labour market, the division of resources within the family, the preponderence of women among single parents and their greater reliance on social security benefits, the fact that women pensioners are more likely to depend on means-tested benefits, all account for women spending a higher proportion of their lives in poverty (Glendinning and Millar, 1987; Payne, 1991). Given the general correlation between poverty and ill health (*Black Report*, 1980), therefore, it is not surprising that—on all measures of ill health—women come off worse than men. Payne concludes from her review of the evidence that women 'experience higher levels of illness than men: women are more likely to report themselves as sick in surveys relying on self-perception as well as those relying on consultation with the medical profession, absenteeism from paid employment and measures of limitation on normal activity' (Payne, 1991: 87.)

There is much evidence that health is related to socio-economic status generally. However, it would also appear that socio-economic status has an impact on the incidence of ill health among women at a younger age than among men. Heyman et al. concluded from their study that 'premature morbidity associated with social class occurs at an earlier age among females than among males and therefore that females are more vulnerable than males to the effects of low social class on long-term health' (Heyman et al., 1990: 181).

While physiological differences may explain some of the differences in levels and cause of impairment found among men and women, gender would appear to be integrally linked to these differences.

Sex, gender and the experience of impairment and disability

Physiological differences between men and women can influence the experience of impairment—what it is like to have a particular impairment. For example, bladder incontinence for spinal-cord injured women is generally recognized to have a more limiting effect on women's lives than it does for spinal-cord injured men because it is physiologically more difficult to deal with bladder incontinence in women. It could be argued, however, that this physiological disadvantage for women has often been compounded by health professionals' failure to help women to deal with incontinence in ways which recognize the reality of their daily lives. A survey of spinal-cord injured women in Britain found, for example, that the method of 'bladder training', which was the most common form of incontinence management offered to women in spinal units up until the mid-1980s, dominated their lives in a way which made daily living very difficult. One woman said, 'It prevents *living* let alone working.' And another said, 'It's the time and effort it takes to cope with this that dominates my life. Bladder training at best only gives me three hours between toilet visits. Compared to a lot of people this is good.' Some women had to express their bladders every hour and a number of women pointed out that each visit was not just a matter of seconds, either. As one said 'I can be on the toilet half an hour or longer' (Morris, 1989).

Since the mid-1980s, spinal units in Britain have tended to change from 'bladder training' to intermittent self-catheterization as a method of incontinence management offered to women. This method most closely copies what the body should do naturally, for all it requires is the insertion of a small catheter each time the bladder needs emptying. Yet the advice offered to women still often tends to restrict their lives in that they are told that, in order to prevent bladder infections, they should not use toilets where they cannot reach the wash-basin while they are sitting on the toilet.

This is an example, not so much of professionals reacting differentially to men and women's needs but to women's needs being different for physiological reasons and professionals failing to give enough thought to the reality of daily life and the consequences of the rehabilitation methods offered.

There are of course other instances in which physiological differences result in particular disadvantages for men. For spinal-cord injured men, for example, the ability to reproduce is much more likely to be affected by their injury than it is for women. Yet the emphasis (and allocation of resources) on infertility is almost entirely on the infertility of non-disabled women. A survey of spinal-cord injured men found that the most frequently mentioned area of unmet need concerned counselling over fertility and sexuality. As one man said, referring to his experience of a spinal unit: 'I came out of there as blank as a dodo—there was never any direct conversation with any of the doctors about fertility—only what you picked up on the ward—no one ever explained that side of it to me—whether I can have kids or anything' (Oliver et al., 1988: 75).

However, while there are these physiological differences which may partly account for some of the different experiences of impairment among men and women, it could be argued that it is predominantly gender—what it is to be a man or woman in our society—which has the bigger influence on men and women's experiences, contributing as it does to the nature of disability, in other words the nature of the experience of exclusion or marginalization. For example, masculinity in western societies is to a large extent defined by physical fitness and the ability to support one's family. An inability to take up paid employment and/or exclusion from the labour market because of direct and indirect discrimination against people with certain types of impairment therefore has a particular impact on men. As Robert Murphy puts it, 'Women *may* work, but men *must* work. And since a large percentage of the motor-disabled are not employed, they are economic dependents, supported by public funds and the incomes of their families. As would be expected, this dependency affects the social standing of men more deeply than women' (Murphy, 1987: 157).

On the other hand, women's social role is predominantly defined by the nurturing tasks that they perform, whether it is caring for young children, running a household, looking after older relatives. These are roles which women who experience impairments perform (Morris, 1993b: chapter 6), although part of the experience of disability is the general assumption that a woman with a significant level of impairment cannot take on a nurturing role, and we will discuss this later when looking at the impact of disability on gender. However, women's caring role—which is such an important part of the social construction of femininity—also has an impact on women's experience of impairment in that these responsibilities inhibit their ability to get their own health-care needs met (Graham, 1990, 1993).

Women's experience of the sexual division of labour within the family can sometimes mean that impairment-related needs are not met. For example, one woman who has multiple sclerosis felt that her condition deteriorated because her husband left all the child care and housework for her to do—'I wanted to leave particularly because MS accelerates with stress and I had a lot of stress. And I was tired out from the work . . . it tired me out.' (Morris, 1993a: 16).

Gender also has an impact on women's experience of disability in that disabled women have higher rates of unemployment (OPCS, 1988b) and are more likely to be on means-tested benefits than disabled men. This is a reflection of the economic inequality experienced by all women. Such inequalities would seem to be particularly apparent among those women who have been disabled for some time. For example, Zarb and Oliver's study of ageing with impairment found that, whereas 48 per cent of the men in their sample had adequate incomes, only 25 per cent of the women did (Zarb and Oliver, 1993: 74).

Gender, impairment and access to services

The way that gender as a social construct influences men and women's experiences can have an impact on whether and how impairment-related needs are responded to by health and social services professionals. Indeed, the very recognition of impairment in men and women is sometimes influenced by gender.

One of the difficulties in measuring impairment and ill health is that conditions or health status in themselves are rarely recorded; rather it is treatments and the use of services which are taken as measurements of impairment and ill health. If the provision and take-up of treatments and services are determined by a variety of social factors (as they are) then the very measurements of ill health and impairment will be social constructs. This is illustrated by the following example.

In the United States during the 1960s men with renal failure on dialysis outnumbered women on dialysis by three to one and it was assumed until the early 1980s that chronic renal failure was more common among men than among women. However, it is now clear that at least half of all renal patients are women and the incidence of chronic renal failure among women is more widely recognized. The change in recognition occurred because, prior to 1972 when Medicare (the American system of subsidized health care) assumed financial responsibility for all dialysis this form of treatment tended to be restricted to people who were young and had few medical complications in addition to their kidney failure. Once greater access to dialysis was assured through Medicare more women got access to this form of treatment and it became clear that the incidence of chronic renal failure among women was about the same as among men. It is not clear whether the previous differential access to dialysis was the result of straightforward sexist assumptions about men being more deserving of treatment (presumably because of their role as breadwinners) or whether the criteria of age and lack of other medical complications indirectly discriminated against women experiencing renal failure (Kutner and Gray, 1985).

This illustrates the important role of health professionals in responding to impairment and the way in which the availability of treatment may be influenced by gender as a social construct. Availability and type of rehabilitation services may also be influenced by gender. For example, rehabilitation services may focus on men's role as paid workers and may fail to respond to their needs as parents. Furthermore, there is considerable evidence that—because rehabilitation services are predominantly concerned with maximizing men's employment opportunities—women's employment needs have not generally been addressed (Lonsdale, 1990).

Gender as a social construct may also influence the way people get access to community-based services. Feminist academics have identified the way that the presence of a non-disabled woman in a household reduces the likelihood of a disabled or older person receiving help from statutory services. Thus, Arber concluded from her analysis of the General Household Survey that 'Disabled women cared for by their husbands are about 20% more likely to receive district nursing support than where a disabled husband is cared for by his wife. Similarly, unmarried sons who care for an elderly parent are about 20% more likely to receive district nursing care than unmarried daughters. Elderly people living with a married child receive the least district nurse support. It is clear that the substitution of informal carers for statutory domestic and personal health services is greater where women are carers' (Arber, 1990: 76).

It must be emphasized that these types of statistics are almost always analysed in terms of the experience of those identified as carers—in this case the 'disadvantaged position of married women who are co-resident with elderly disabled people' (Arber, 1990: 78). It is also clear, however, that the gender of the disabled person is related to whether statutory help is provided. For example, the same General Household Survey indicated that older women living alone are less likely to receive either home helps or district nursing services than men living alone (Arber, 1990: 77).

Moreover, we need to know whether such differential access to district nursing and other services is part of a disadvantaged experience for disabled people and in order to answer this we need to know whether disabled people who receive, for example, district nursing services are more advantaged than those who do not. There has been much written about the 'burden' experienced by those identified as informal carers and the restrictions on their lives but very little about the experience of disabled people in terms of the comparison between receiving help from family and friends, from statutory services and from those employed by disabled people themselves (although see Zarb and Oliver, 1993, Morris, 1993a and b).

Disability and the experience of men and women

Disability, masculinity and femininity

Just as sex and gender can be shown to influence the experience of impairment and disability so can impairment and disability influence the experience of being a man or a woman. Indeed, social attitudes towards impairment can influence whether disabled people are treated as men or women at all. Michelene Mason's account of how the people around her as she grew up assumed that she would not experience the physical and social consequences of being female is a familiar experience for people who are born with an impairment.

> In retrospect I think it is quite amazing, although I did not realise it at the time, that in the whole of my childhood I can only remember one reference to my future adult life. This was a conversation between myself, my sister then aged about 12, and my mother. I cannot remember the origins of the subject, but a remark was made about my sister becoming an aunty. Her response was, 'Oh yes, and *who* is going to make me an aunty?' My mother said 'Sssh!' and that was it—that was the only time my future adult life was ever referred to.

I was not told by my immediate family about menstruation even when it happened. I think, in fact they were quite surprised that it did happen.

[She went away to Florence Treloars Grammar School for Physically Disabled Girls at the age of 14.]

> Our academic abilities were nurtured very well compared to our previous experiences of so-called 'Special Education', but even here was the unspoken expectation that work would be 'instead of' the usual expectations of women—not only to work but also to get married and have a family. Our sexuality was barely acknowledged by the staff. We did not have any sex education. (Mason, 1992: 114)

Similarly, many disabled men—particularly those born with an impairment or who acquire it in childhood or early adulthood—find that the social roles which non-disabled men take for granted are not open to them. The importance of these roles for their sense of self-esteem is illustrated by the experience of one man whose initial experience of disability was that of being confined within residential care and of having no social role other than that of a dependant. However, after he and another resident fell in love, married and set up home together, he said:

> I'm a husband, a father and a breadwinner. And ten years ago I was in an institution where I couldn't even decide when I would go to the toilet . . . you know, you can't really understand it if you haven't done it . . . your whole life changes. (Morris 1993a: 30)

Becoming a mother or a father is an important part of being a man or a woman in our society and to be denied such an opportunity has serious consequences for someone's social role and also their self-identity. Men and women who have learning difficulties are often denied the opportunity to be parents. Women, in particular, 'have their sexuality carefully policed so that they do not become pregnant' (Walmsley, 1993: 133). Motherhood is a very important part of the caring role which women have in western society and women with learning difficulties who are denied this opportunity often feel bereft. The pain is particularly acute for those whose children are taken away from them. One black woman whom Walmsley interviewed had her daughter taken into care at the age of two and expressed a longing to have her back:

> The only child I've got you know. I'd like to have her back, look after her hair, plait her hair and oil it cos she can't do that . . . her skin is dry now. I liked cooking for her you know, like baked potatoes, rice, minced beef, I did all that . . . (1993: 134)

Disability and men and women's access to services

The experience of disability—social attitudes towards impairment and the general exclusion from the mainstream—can influence men and women's access to services. For example, attitudes held about disabled people can influence a man or a woman's access to contraceptive advice. Those who have visible mobility and/or communication impairments, particularly those who are wheelchair users, are commonly perceived to be asexual, partly because assumptions are held that no one would find them sexually attractive, partly because disabled people are often treated as children.

Amongst the 205 spinal-cord injured women who participated in the *Able Lives* survey, the most common experience was of a lack of advice about contraception following injury. While things may have improved in spinal units, women injured in the mid-1980s still found, as one tersely said, 'No advice of this nature has ever been given by anyone' (Morris, 1989: 93). Women had similar experiences with their GPs: as one woman said, 'I was never given any advice on which type of contraceptive to use because I think my doctor thought that because of my paralysis I shouldn't need any birth control' (1989: 93). Among those who did receive advice, different information was given about using the pill. Some were told that the pill was the best form of contraception for them while others were told that there was a risk of thrombosis among spinal-cord injured women and that therefore they should avoid this form of contraception. One woman said, 'The family planning clinics in my county know little about disabled women and very few disabled women go to them' (1989: 94); this may well at least partly account for such contradictory advice.

Little is written about disabled men and women's access to health services such as family planning, infertility clinics, breast and cervical cancer screening, maternity services and so on. On the other hand, there is much anecdotal evidence about poor physical access, a dearth of information in accessible formats (tape, large print, Braille, sign) and a general assumption held by many health professionals that disabled people are not part of the general public for whom mainstream services are provided.

Women who have significant physical impairments and need help with daily living activities often experience great difficulty in getting help with the tasks which are part of being a mother. If a woman is physically to look after a small child and not have to hand this responsibility over to someone else, it is necessary for her to be able to direct the personal assistance she requires. This is rarely possible if she is dependent on statutory services and help received from a partner or parent may well interfere with her own relationship with her child. As one woman, married with one child, said,

> I first got P.A.s [personal assistants who she employs herself] when Molly was very small . . . I didn't want my mother doing the things that I would have done . . . I didn't want Molly running to her instead of to me and it would have been difficult for her to stop that happening if at the same time she was going to have a normal relationship as a grand-mother to Molly. So that's when I got the money off the Council to employ people and I could tell them exactly what to do . . . you know, like if she fell over and hurt herself then they were to pick her up and put her on my lap so it was me that did the kissing better. And of course Molly was fond of my P.A.s but it was always clear that I was her mother. (Morris, 1993b: 91–92)

Unfortunately, many disabled women who rely on statutory ser-vices find that they cannot get help with the tasks that are part of being a mother: for example, one woman—parenting within a lesbian rela-tionship—found that she could only get help with personal care tasks and not the physical help that she needed to look after a 2 year old. She talked about how:

> The thing I was upset about is just the fact that we're [she and her partner] so glued together. Like my relationship with Dan [the 2 year old] is practically totally dependent on Ros so my ability to have separate time, a separate relationship with Dan is not there, and Ros' ability to have her own life is pretty non-existent as well. (Morris, 1993b: 82)

A very important part of the oppression which disabled people experience is the way that the social consequences of impairment influence their experience as men and women—whether they get their needs met as men and women and whether they can take on the social roles associated with being a man or a woman.

Conclusion

Disability is an experience of inequality but the nature of this experi-ence is also influenced by other social inequalities: class and race being two important influences which we have not discussed in this chap-ter. In order to understand fully the experience of disability it is necessary to consider the interaction between gender and disability as social constructs as well as their interaction with the bodily char-acteristics of sex and impairment. Much work remains to be done in exploring these relationships, making sense of disabled men and women's experiences and challenging both oppressive stereotypes and unequal access to services.

References

Arber, S. (1990) Revealing women's health: re-analysing the General Household Survey. In *Women's Health Counts* (ed. H. Roberts), Routledge, London, 63–92

Arber, S. and Ginn, J. (1991) *Gender and Later Life*, Sage, London

Black Report (1980), Report of the working party on inequalities in health, chaired by Sir Douglas Black, Department of Health and Social Security, London

Glendinning, C. and Millar, J. (eds) (1987) *Women and Poverty in Britain*, Harvester Wheatsheaf, Hemel Hempstead

Graham, H. (1990) Behaving well: women's health behaviour in context. In *Women's Health Counts* (ed. H. Roberts), Routledge, London, 195–219

Graham, H. (1993) *Hardship and Health in Women's Lives*, Harvester Wheatsheaf, Hemel Hempstead

Hanna, J. H. and Rogovsky, B. (1991) Women with disabilities: two handicaps plus. *Disability Handicap and Society*, **6 (1)**, 49–64

Hart, N. (1989), Sex, gender and survival: inequalities of life chances between European men and women. In *Health Inequalities in European Countries* (ed J. Fox), Gower, Aldershot, 64–79

Heyman, B. et al. (1990) Social class and the prevalence of handicapping conditions. *Disability, Handicap and Society*, **5, (2)** 167–184

Kutner, N. and Gray, H. (1985) Women and chronic renal failure: some neglected issues. In *Women and Disability: The Double Handicap* (ed. M. J. Deegan and N. A. Brooks), Transaction Books, New Brunswick, USA, 105–116

Lonsdale, S. (1990) *Women and Disability*, Macmillan, London

Mason, M. (1992) A nineteen parent family. In *Alone Together: Voices of Single Mothers*, (ed. J. Morris), The Women's Press, London, 112–125

Morris, J. (ed.) (1989) *Able Lives: Women's Experience of Paralysis*, The Women's Press, London

Morris, J. (1993a) *Community Care or Independent Living*, Joseph Rowntree Foundation, York

Morris, J. (1993b) *Independent Lives? Community Care and Disabled People*, Macmillan, Basingstoke

Murphy, R. (1987) *The Body Silent*, J. M. Dent & Sons, London

Oliver, M. et al. (1988) *Walking into Darkness: The Experience of Spinal Cord Injury*, Macmillan, Basingstoke

OPCS (1988a) *The Prevalence of Disability among Adults*, Office of Population Censuses and Surveys, London

OPCS (1988b) *The Financial Circumstances of Disabled Adults Living in Private Households*, Office of Population Censuses and Surveys, London

Patrick, D. L. (1989) Screening for disability. In *Disablement in the Community* (ed. D. L. Patrick and H. Peach) Oxford Medical Publications, Oxford, 19–38

Payne, S. (1991) *Women, Health and Poverty*, Harvester Wheatsheaf, Hemel Hempstead

Walmsley, J. (1993) Contradictions in caring: reciprocity and interdependence. *Disability Handicap and Society*, **8, 2**, 129–142

Zarb, G. and Oliver, M. (1993) *Ageing with a Disability: What do They Expect After all These Years?* University of Greenwich, London

16

Disabled health and welfare professionals

Sally French

It is frequently argued that having personal experience of an event gives a dimension of knowledge that others cannot fully share. Childbirth is an example of this, where mothers may assume that neither men nor childless women can fully appreciate the experience. Various self-help groups have been formed because of dissatisfaction with the help that professionals provide or a realization that such help is limited. Many believe that minority group members have better insight, more commitment and greater rapport with similarly affected people than does the general population (Shearer, 1981; Wainapel, 1987), and that people with extensive professional training do not necessarily help those who are disabled (McKnight, 1981).

Disabled people are widely discriminated against in most types of employment which makes it likely that they will find entry to high status professions, such as the health and welfare professions, particularly difficult. In a content analysis of the career literature of 26 health and welfare professions and occupations, it was found that disabled people were never specifically invited to apply, yet ten of these occupations explicitly sought candidates with the ability to empathize and understand ill and disabled people (French, 1986). The radiography profession, for example, was seeking people with tact and empathy (College of Radiographers, 1985) and the audiology technician was required to have 'a sympathetic and understanding personality' (British Society of Audiology). These are qualities which disabled people, by virtue of their experiences, are likely to possess. Burnfield, a psychiatrist with multiple sclerosis states:

> I believe that having MS has helped me to become more sensitive to the needs of others and that it has enhanced my skills as a healer. I often think of myself as being doubly qualified, firstly as a patient and secondly as a doctor—the order is important. (1985: 169)

Similarly, a blind physiotherapist said:

The frustrations of disability are much the same in as much as it is a physical limitation on your life and you think 'if only'. . . . Having to put up with that for so long I know ever so well what patients mean when they mention those kinds of difficulties. (French 1990a: 1)

Stetten, a visually-impaired physician, is concerned about the narrowness of ophthalmologists' interests. He claimed to have learned far more about visual impairment from chance contact with other visually-impaired people, and believes that ophthalmologists have come to confine their real interest in medicine 'to events which occur within the globe of the eye' (1983: 27).

It is not uncommon for disabled people to complain about the treatment and lack of understanding they receive at the hands of health and welfare professionals; a disabled person featured in Sutherland's book recalls her contact with medical personnel as 'a whole series of experiences of being very coldly and formally mauled around' (1981: 123). Similarly, a nurse with epilepsy states 'It seemed to me that the doctors and nurses looking after me had a most appalling lack of insight into the problems of a patient with epilepsy' (Campling 1981: 61).

Attitudes towards disabled workers

In a review of the literature concerning the employment of disabled people, there is considerable evidence to show that they are as productive and efficient as non-disabled workers (Kettle, 1979). Disabled people are also less likely to have accidents or be absent from work than their non-disabled peers (Darnbrough and Kinrade, 1981; Local Government Management Board, 1991). This information is, however, largely unknown or ignored and disabled people are frequently assumed to be less capable than other workers, to be absent more often and to be more accident prone (Kettle, 1979).

Similarly, most of the overt justification for the exclusion of disabled people from the health and welfare professions is in terms of the disabled people themselves; their presumed inability to cope, the adverse effect they may have on patients and clients, and the assumption of proneness to accidents (Browning, 1980; Chickadonz, 1983; Libman, 1983). Not all health and welfare professionals subscribe to these views, however. Many people have expressed the view that disabled people have unique assets to offer the health and welfare professions (Hutchins, 1978; Biehn, 1979; Gavin, 1980; Bueche, 1983; Turner, 1984; Wainapel, 1987; Teager, 1987; O'Hare and Thomson, 1991), and studies carried out by the American Society of Handicapped Physicians show that approximately 75 per cent of doctors with a wide variety of impairments, remain successfully employed in clinical practice (Wainapel and Bernbaum, 1986; Wainapel, 1987). Turner notes the hypocrisy of excluding disabled people from the health and welfare professions. He states:

> How can we tell patients they can lead normal lives when we don't allow their peers to become our colleagues? Though not yet illegal to discriminate on health grounds, there can be no doubt that it is immoral and unethical to do so. (1984: 451)

French (1987) found that the attitudes of physiotherapists towards hypothetical people with various impairments appeared to be similar to those of the general public; for example when asked which people would be suitable candidates for physiotherapy education, they were far more positive towards those with controlled diabetes than those with controlled epilepsy, and were doubtful about people who had experienced mental illness. It is even possible that the views of health and welfare professionals are more negative than those of the general public due to the type of relationship they have with disabled people, and the fact that they come into contact only when disabled people are most in need of help.

Prolonged contact with disabled people as colleagues may have some effect on the attitudes of non-disabled professionals. Visually-impaired people have been part of the physiotherapy profession since 1915; in a study by French (1987) they were viewed as more suitable for the work, by non-disabled physiotherapists, than people with most other impairments. Weller and Grunes (1988) point out that contact with disabled people breaks down stereotypical categories. Despite this acceptance, there is little evidence that the profession has accommodated substantially to their needs in either employment or educational practice (French, 1990b; French, in progress). Indeed Teager goes as far as to remark, 'The general acceptance of the blind physiotherapist has been hard won, is difficult to preserve, and will be constantly subject to the closest scrutiny' (1987: 135).

Negative attitudes are sometimes rationalized and disguised as concern, emphasizing that disabled people may damage themselves, by undertaking such demanding work (Safilios-Rothschild, 1976; French, 1986). Many sociologists have commented on the paternalism of medical practice (Faulder, 1985), and Sutherland (1981) notes that professionals base their dealings on a dependency model in which they are the experts and people who are disabled are dependent on them for help. When discussing the issue of disabled people becoming health professionals he states 'Since the job for which the person is applying would confer a recognition of equality, they tend not to get it, they are judged unsuitable' (1981: 40). Chinnery (1991) points out that there are far fewer disabled people employed in the health and welfare services in the United Kingdom than the government's recommended quota of 3 per cent, and that most of those who are employed manage to 'pass' as non-disabled people.

There is other evidence to suggest that the health and welfare professions have not been particularly positive in their attitudes towards disabled people, nor knowledgeable about the implications of disability. For example in the 1984 career literature of the Chartered Society of Physiotherapy it is stated:

> Any form of physical disability or weakness is likely to contra-indicate physiotherapy as a suitable career, in particular defects in hearing, epilepsy, chest ailments, skin conditions, heart defects, nervous break-downs. Injuries to backs, knees and hands may also prejudice acceptance for training. (Chartered Society of Physiotherapy, 1984: 2)

Similarly the Royal College of Nursing (1985) believes that candidates with a variety of medical conditions and characteristics, including obesity, eczema and amputations, are unsuitable for training. Such statements show the most blatant form of negative discrimination, implying that subtler forms also exist. It should be remembered, however, that attitudes and practice have undergone considerable change in the past few years, and that the views put forward by professional bodies do not necessarily reflect the views of their memberships.

Moon (1990) carried out a study of twelve nurses who became disabled, only four of whom were still employed. She found their experiences very mixed but overall the help they received was inadequate and patchy. There was disagreement between the disabled nurses and their employers in 50 per cent of cases about whether the disability would affect their ability to work. Craik (1990) asserts, however, that the profession of occupational therapy welcomes disabled applicants and that their numbers are increasing.

Goffman (1968) believes that disabled people have a discredited social identity whereby their disability becomes their 'master status' obscuring all other attributes. He believes that those who associate closely with disabled people on an equal basis are likely to acquire a 'courtesy stigma' whereby they become 'contaminated' themselves. This detraction of image may be a further reason why disabled people are not accepted in the health and welfare professions in greater numbers.

Disabled people are often viewed as weak and ineffective which contradicts the popular image of a health or welfare professional. Young, for example, believes that patients view their doctors as 'God-like figures; strong, powerful, clever and in control of some kind of magic' (1981: 153). Perhaps it is the health and welfare professionals, however, who depend on this image more than the patients or clients, as a strategy to obscure their real lack of power in the face of illness, disability and death, as well as serving to enhance the placebo effect. These feelings are captured in the Biblical quotation, 'Physician heal thyself' (Luke 4, verse 23), the implications being that physicians who are powerless to escape disability and illness are unlikely to have the ability to heal or to help others. There is, however, an ancient maxim that 'only the wounded physician heals' (Bennet, 1987: 206); it is a common belief that the only way to gain full understanding of an event or situation is to experience it first hand.

Many beliefs about disability are irrational and date back to ancient times. Disability and illness have been associated with punishment, evil and sin (Foucault, 1967; Helman, 1984). Such images are plentiful in the Bible, in drama, film and literature (Rieser, 1992a; 1992b; Cumberbatch and Negrine, 1992). It is possible that some of these perceptions, being part of our culture, may colour professional attitudes, albeit sub-consciously. Some researchers have found, however, that it is disruption to social interaction, rather than attribution of responsibility, which appears to explain the social distance from individuals with various impairments (Albrecht, 1982). The need for effective social interaction and good communication skills is strongly emphasized by many of the health and welfare professions, and the belief that disabled people lack these skills may serve as a powerful justification for their exclusion.

In contrast, disability is sometimes romanticized and associated with goodness, or disabled people may be perceived as having more insight or greater perception than others. In a questionnaire study of the attitudes of physiotherapists to the recruitment of disabled people into that profession (French, 1987), it was found that twenty subjects (10 per cent) believed that visually-impaired physiotherapists have greater powers of touch, with a further seven subjects (3 per cent), believing that their perceptiveness in general is enhanced.

In another study where visually-impaired physiotherapists were interviewed (French, 1990a), many reported that their patients had mystical beliefs about them, for example that they had a 'sixth sense' or a refined sense of touch. Some of the physiotherapists tried to dispel these misconceptions, while others regarded them as beneficial both in terms of the placebo effect and, for those in private practice, in terms of business. One physiotherapist said:

> Patients do have this feeling that there is this extra magical quality. . . . Even though this is an illusion, why not use it to advantage? Although we are physiotherapists I think we are quite often psychotherapists as well, and if we can utilise something like that I'm not opposed to doing so if it achieves a good result in the end. (French 1990a:3)

Mystical beliefs about disabled people may assist them in their quest to become health and welfare professionals, although an unfortunate side effect of such beliefs is the assumption that disabled people need no specific help or consideration. Such beliefs can, in fact, conveniently serve to deny disabled people the assistance they require.

It is unclear whether disabled people are actively discouraged from entering the health and welfare professions, but it seems likely that the acceptance of more than a few could seriously challenge the traditional professional/client relationship where the professional is considered to be the expert and occupies a dominant position over the client. Sociologists and disabled people alike have written extensively of the conflicts in the professional/client relationship which often seem to arise through differing conceptions and definitions of illness and disability (Scott, 1969; Morris, 1989). Sutherland (1981) notes that disabled people are likely to possess skills which non-disabled people lack, yet in order to improve these skills professionals would need to learn from their disabled clients which, in turn, would lead to a reduction in their own authority and status.

Professional etiquette has been described as a body of ritual which preserves before the client the common front of the profession (Hughes, 1946). Goffman (1969) notes that intimate co-operation is required if a given projected definition is to be maintained, and that teams will only recruit people who can be trusted to perform 'correctly'; thus professionals tend to select recruits 'in their own image' admitting only those who are likely to conform with values considered to be important to the profession.

There is much evidence to suggest that disability may be just one attribute which is considered undesirable in members of the health and welfare professions; race and class discrimination are well documented (Cole, 1987; Pearson, 1987; Baxter, 1988) and gender discrimination is also marked (Young, 1981). In addition French (1986) found that various characteristics which go against the stereotyped image of the physiotherapist are stigmatized by that profession; for example, to be very overweight was considered more of a barrier than blindness or using a wheelchair. The social acceptability of a disability may, therefore, be more important than the limitations to which it may give rise.

A further factor which may exclude disabled people from the health and welfare professions is that of social class (Young, 1981; Watkins, 1987). Although the situation is changing, health and welfare professionals tend to come from middle-class backgrounds (Young, 1981; Scrivens, 1982), whereas the majority of disabled people come from working-class homes (Smith and Jacobson, 1988). Goffman (1969) believes that in order to maintain their status and power, professionals need to keep a certain distance between themselves and their clients, thus a professional member of less power and status may be perceived as a threat. He states 'If the team is to maintain the impression that it is fostering then there must be some assurance that no individual will be allowed to join both team and audience,' (1969: 97). Yet by definition a disabled health or welfare professional would belong to both groups. (For a more detailed discussion of the relationship between disabled people and health and welfare professionals, the reader is referred to chapter 8.)

Sutherland (1981) believes that the stigma of low socio-economic class is added to that of disability and, conversely, that a middle class background may serve to reduce the stigma of disability. He explains:

> It is much easier to counteract the stereotyped ideas about disability on which discrimination is based if one possesses a middle-class background and accent, a university education and the particular type of articulacy and confidence that these factors produce. (1981: 35)

There has been very little research specifically addressing the perceptions and experiences of disabled health and welfare professionals. Because of the paucity of research in this area, the rest of this chapter will examine a small study of 25 health and welfare professionals, who were accepted for professional education despite substantial disabilities (French, 1988).

Method and procedure

In this study 25 disabled people currently employed or training in the health and welfare professions were interviewed, and one person, who was working abroad, sent a written account of her experiences using the interview schedule as a guide. The sample consisted of nine men and sixteen women and represented seven professions and seventeen types of impairment; two people had dual qualifications. All but two of the interviewees were accepted for professional education as disabled people, the others acquired their impairments during training; ten people had trained within the past five years and fourteen within the past ten years. The professions and impairments represented are shown in Table 16.1.

Locating these people was difficult and the interviewing involved travelling as far north as Dundee and as far west as Exeter. This, in itself, gives some indication that the recruitment of substantially disabled people into these professions is unusual. The interviews were semi-structured but the respondents were encouraged to expand their ideas freely. The interviews lasted between 15 and 90 minutes, with all but two being tape-recorded; they were then transcribed and the information was categorized by the researcher by

Table 16.1

Professions	Number
Medicine	4
Physiotherapy	7
Occupational therapy	3
Social work	4
Nurse/nurse tutor	1
Prosthetics	3
Counselling	2
Occupational therapy/physiotherapy	1
	25

Impairments	
Visual impairment	4
Cerebral palsy	1
Cerebral palsy/visual impairment	1
Cerebral palsy/hearing impairment	1
Lower limb amputation	4
Tetraplegia	1
Multiple sclerosis	1
Epilepsy	1
Ileostomy	1
Achondroplasia	1
Hearing disability	3
Shoulder/cervical abnormalities	1
Recurrent dislocation of patella	1
Rheumatoid arthritis	1
Ankylosing spondylitis	1
Spina bifida	1
Liver disease	1
	25

means of content analysis. The researcher's own visual impairment was disclosed to aid communication and reduce suspicion.

Findings

Perceived advantages and disadvantages of being a disabled health or welfare professional

All the disabled professionals could see advantages relating to being disabled in the work context. The most common response was that they felt better able to empathize with their patients and clients and understand the social and psychological implications of disability.

Most felt they could empathize with and understand those with a similar impairment best. A partially-deaf therapist stated 'I've got a lot more patience with deaf people and I get more out of them. The doctors say "forget it, ask a relative" but I speak to them.' All the deaf people found the ability to lip read helpful. One mentioned her skill at communicating with patients with tracheostomies, and another found she could lip read patients when nobody else could understand them. One spoke sign language fluently and was sometimes used as an interpreter.

Most of the disabled professionals believed they had more knowledge of disability than their colleagues. A prosthetist who had a lower-limb amputation himself stated 'They (patients) want to pick your brain for every bit of knowledge they can get. They're very interested to find out how you coped.' He found he was able to identify patients' problems, especially the small, less obvious ones which other prosthetists might miss or regard as trivial.

Many reported that their patients and clients frequently commented on the advantage of the disability from their own point of view. A prosthetist with an amputation himself remarked, 'Patients say, "you've got one, you know what I mean" '. Similarly a doctor said 'Very many people have told me they can talk to me because I know what it feels like to have an illness. Once you get over that hump of being accepted (for training) then you can use your disability.' Many people found that being disabled helped to break down professional barriers. A deaf therapist said 'They don't see me as a health professional who knows it all who doesn't really understand, they see me as a disabled person.' A doctor found the patients' interest in his electric wheelchair useful in this respect, and a social worker found his guide dog helped, he remarked 'Even when there's an awful atmosphere he's wagging his tail. He's definitely an ice breaker.'

Several people spoke of the advantage of needing help from their patients or clients. A counsellor explained, 'By me needing help it's actually saying "This is a partnership" '. Similarly a blind social worker commented 'I'm able to say to my clients, "I'll help you but there are certain ways in which you are going to have to help me", and the client doesn't feel totally taken over or totally worthless'.

Some people mentioned that they acted as models to their patients or clients showing them what could be achieved; a doctor reported that patients would say, 'I'm off work with a sore knee and there you are working on your crutches.' Several people mentioned that fellow students had learned a great deal about all aspects of disability through having them in the peer group. A therapist with rheumatoid arthritis recalled how annoyed her fellow students became when a lecturing consultant spoke of one of his patients as 'My little RA girl'.

Many people had been asked to counsel patients or clients who were similarly disabled, or to demonstrate their ability to cope. Several people said they had been asked to lecture to a wide range of students and colleagues on the subject of their particular impairment, or on disability in general. A number of the disabled professionals were actively involved in disability issues; several had written books and articles and others were involved in voluntary work. Some had given radio talks and one had founded a society for people with his own impairment.

Some people pointed out that patients and clients who enjoy being in the sick or disabled role could find the disabled health or welfare professional problematic. This can be viewed as a disadvantage from the patient's or client's point of view but perhaps as an advantage from a professional standpoint in that pressure is put on the patient or client to comply.

Many people felt that the advantages of being disabled not only cancelled out any disadvantages there might be but actually outweighed them. A doctor commented 'MS has been something I've used. Having MS has been an added dimension in my training, in my understanding of people, and in the development of my expertise and skills', and a prosthetist said 'You have a great understanding of their problems because no matter how good a prosthetist is, if he's got two legs he falls short of really knowing what it's like.' However, two of the disabled professionals firmly believed that being disabled gave them no additional insight into disability, and one person with a congenital impairment said she had no special understanding of acquired disability.

Some people pointed out the advantages of their work from a personal point of view. Several physiotherapists mentioned that the active nature of the job benefited them physically, and a number of people with sensory impairments believed the nature of the work prevented them from becoming isolated. A profoundly-deaf therapist said 'I do feel that if I didn't have this type of job where I'm meeting different people every day I would withdraw very quickly into myself.'

A few of the disabled professionals pointed out the disadvantages that could arise as a result of being disabled when interacting with patients or clients. A few people found that being disabled had the effect of trivializing the patients' or clients' problems. A doctor found that his severe disability inhibited psychiatric patients from discussing their difficulties, and a psychiatrist found that some of his patients had a tendency to mother him and could find it difficult in psychoanalysis to express anger or hostility for fear that it would 'damage' him in some way. An occupational therapist found that elderly confused patients occasionally lacked confidence in her but she managed the situation by reassuring them and immediately focusing attention back on them.

A blind person found lack of non-verbal communication a problem, though others felt able to compensate and even viewed blindness as helpful in some situations. For example, a social worker felt that clients could speak more honestly to him because they knew he could not recognize them in other contexts, and a counsellor reported that clients found her blindness helped them to speak more openly. The prosthetists with amputations noted that patients could be discouraged by seeing them cope so well. They would sometimes say, 'If only I could walk like you.' The prosthetists were, however, acutely aware of this and were very careful never to compare themselves with their patients.

Access to professional education

Of the 23 disabled professionals who had been accepted for professional education as disabled people, eight reported that their entry qualifications were better than average, and five thought that this was a major factor in their acceptance for professional education. A further eight people said they had been helped to gain access to professional education by an influential person. Such people were either doctors of high status who knew the individual personally, or someone on the selection panel with particular knowledge or interest in disability, for example a person interviewing a blind candidate had a visually-impaired son. Twelve people felt that their acceptance for professional education had been strongly influenced by one of these two factors. In addition a doctor mentioned the advantage of his socially privileged background, and several people indicated that they came from 'medical' families.

All but one person revealed their impairments before the selection interview. Several, especially those with relatively hidden impairments, were uncertain of the wisdom of this and spoke of being in a dilemma over the issue. A profoundly-deaf person felt it was best to reveal her disability after contact had been made because of the 'funny ideas' people have about deafness.

Of the 23 health and welfare professionals who were accepted for professional education as disabled people, eight experienced difficulty. An occupational therapist stated, 'It didn't matter what I said, they said I couldn't cope', and a physiotherapist recalled, 'His parting words were "nobody will accept you as a physio, no school's going to accept you." ' Interestingly she was later accepted by the very person who had said this! Several people mentioned that getting as far as the interview was the main problem, a counsellor concluded that professionals 'Have conditioned themselves to believing that the disabled person is the person who should be helped rather than the helper.'

Some people were turned down by one college on the grounds of disability, but were willingly accepted by another. Several people who were refused entry to physiotherapy education because of disability gained access to occupational therapy without difficulty, and one person who was told by her school career service that every type of work involving patients would be out of the question, was accepted into pharmacy, nursing and physiotherapy. It must be emphasized, however, that the majority of the disabled professionals, 15 of the 23, experienced no problems regarding their acceptance for professional education.

Attitudes of teachers

Some people experienced negative attitudes from their teachers. The most common complaint was a general lack of adaptation to meet their needs. A physiotherapist recalled 'They weren't obstructive, but they didn't go out of their way to be helpful either', and a deaf therapist said 'I couldn't follow the lectures at all, yet I didn't feel I could keep saying "I'm deaf, will you look at me." ' Some felt they were viewed in terms of being disabled, while others mentioned that their teachers lacked confidence in them. Several blind people complained of the excessive concern over their inability to make eye contact with clients and the difficulty they had convincing teaching staff that they could cope. A blind social worker said 'They concentrated an awful lot on silly things. There was no comment at all about whether I'd be able to cope with the course, they were concentrating on whether I'd be able to find my way from the station.'

A doctor who acquired his impairment during training felt unable to confide in the staff. He stated:

> I was very frightened that if I had a disease like that they might suggest that I wasn't able to continue the training and that I wouldn't qualify. I felt if I mentioned them (the symptoms) they'd think I was skiving, or malingering or being a hypochondriac or neurotic, and I wasn't going to be labelled as those things.

Similarly, a physiotherapist said 'I had to try and keep a brave face on it and not let on, I thought it might affect my career, they might just chuck me out.'

Only two of the 25 disabled professionals were given substantial concessions during their professional education. Some people were openly informed that there would be no special help. A deaf therapist said 'They felt that if I wanted to be on the course, I'd got to manage the same as everyone else. The foreign students got more help.' Their feelings about concessions were, however, mixed. A blind person remarked 'If someone said to me "You'd better not do this placement" then I'd rather walk to Australia on my hands than admit that I couldn't.'

Despite these various difficulties, only six people failed to complete their courses in the minimum possible time.

Twelve of the disabled professionals could recall negative attitudes from their teachers, although they all related instances of positive attitudes too. The remaining 13 regarded the attitudes of their teachers as either neutral or good. A physiotherapist said that she could not recall any aggravation at any level, and an occupational therapist stated 'It didn't matter what problems I had, I just had to go to them and they'd say "OK, there's a way round it." '

Employment

The attitudes of colleagues were reported as being overwhelmingly good, although a few people mentioned a certain lack of understanding, saying that their colleagues tended to forget or deny that they were disabled which could create difficulties. For example a deaf therapist said that people forgot to look at her when speaking, and a blind social worker said that certain colleagues felt snubbed when he did not respond to their smiles and waves. A person with epilepsy found that sometimes people did not believe what she said, and in one job she was suspected of theft when items went missing. Some people said they had really to press for what they needed; a visually-impaired social worker had to fight for an office where he could adjust the lighting and get away from colleagues who were so fascinated by his visual aids that he could not get on with his work! Several people said that colleagues failed to realize that to produce the same quantity and quality of work, it was necessary to work both harder and longer.

Both during their education and after qualifying some people said they had been encouraged by senior colleagues to work with disabled people, or in areas of medicine considered to be of low prestige. A blind person was accepted for a post on the condition that initially he would work with blind clients. A counsellor commented, 'They always assumed I'd do disability counselling, they were hanging a label round my neck.' A physiotherapist was asked, 'Don't you think you should be working with the young chronic sick?' and an occupational therapist was advised to work in psychiatry. After successfully qualifying, two people were advised by members of their own profession to do full-time voluntary work. Some people decided to work with those with the same type of impairment as themselves. This could lead to suspicion: two people complained that colleagues thought they might 'over-identify' thereby lacking objectivity.

Most people, however, had met with very positive attitudes at work. A deaf therapist commented, 'I depend a little on the staff but they never seem to mind, they never force me into anything.' Only three people reported any instances of negative attitudes from patients or clients.

Just four of the disabled professionals had difficulty finding work. However, a few did meet with negative attitudes in the process. At her first interview in a large London teaching hospital, an occupational therapist was told: 'I must be perfectly honest, I don't see any point in showing you round.' One problem encountered was the expectation in some of these professions that newly-qualified staff should 'rotate' to different medical specialities thereby gaining varied experience, a practice not possible for all the disabled professionals. Some people observed that working in senior posts was easier. A deaf person spoke extensively of the advantages of being in charge. She explained 'I'm the boss and I delegate what I can't do. I'm in control and I know what's going on, all communication comes through me.'

Many people felt that in order to cope, both during professional education and at work, it was necessary to work harder and be more determined, they spoke of a need to 'prove' themselves. A prosthetist said 'You've got to keep up with the fellow next to you and be better than him. You've got to work harder at it because there's a weakness there and that's what they'll play on.' Others had come to the conclusion, however, that these feelings originated from within themselves: a blind person had started to ask himself, 'To whom am I proving what?'

Where possible people tended to specialize early. They tried to find work where they could function well, for example a deaf person said she would avoid a position which involved treating patients in groups, and would never work in a very large hospital. However, people with the same type of impairment had differing views concerning the suitability or unsuitability of various areas of work; this seemed to be due both to the severity of the impairment and to personality factors, it would therefore seem unwise to generalize.

Fifteen of the disabled professionals were restricted in the type of work they could do. For example the doctor who used crutches said he would find surgery difficult and could not visit patients at home because of access problems. However, by choosing their specialities and places of work carefully, most people reported that they could fulfil all of their work obligations.

Conclusion

The findings of this research show that the majority of the disabled professionals had received positive treatment from teachers, colleagues, clients and patients during their professional education and at work. A sizable minority, however, had experienced some degree of negative discrimination, either as a result of work structures or their colleagues' attitudes and lack of understanding. Most of these problems occurred when attempting to gain access to, and during, professional education. At this time disabled individuals have no professional status themselves the possession of which may serve to reduce the stigma of disability after they have qualified. The inequalities inherent in the teacher/student relationship may also create a situation where negative attitudes can be expressed more readily, especially as the educational structures of many of these professions have, until fairly recently, been highly authoritarian.

The degree of discrimination against disabled people working in the health and welfare professions cannot be assessed by this research. It also remains unclear to what extent disabled people have a better understanding of illness and disability than their non-disabled colleagues; it can be argued, however, that this is a redundant issue as disabled people should not be expected to perform at a higher level than others in order to be accepted.

It is evident that further research is needed in this little researched area. This small study does, however, suggest that disabled professionals are no less capable than their non-disabled colleagues and that they may have unique assets to bring to these professions. The implementation of innovative equal opportunities policies which address physical, structural and attitudinal barriers in the workplace, such as the inaccessibility of learning opportunities and the necessity for disabled staff to 'rotate', could go a long way towards helping disabled people realize their full potential as health and welfare professionals.

References

Ability Counts (1991) Local Government Management Board, London

Albrecht, G. (1982) Social distance from the stigmatised: a test of two theories. *Social Science and Medicine,* **16**, 1319–1327

Baxter, C. (1988) *The Black Nurse: An Endangered Species,* National Extension College for Training in Health and Race, London

Bennet, G. (1987) *The Wound of the Doctor,* Secker & Warburg, London

Biehn, J. (1979) Psychiatric illness in physicians. *Journal of the Canadian Medical Association*, **2**, 1342

British Society of Audiology (undated), *Employment and Training of Audiology Technicians*, London

Browning, H. K. E. (1980) Careers for diabetic girls in nursing. *British Medical Journal*, **255**, 307.

Bueche, M. S. (1983) Student with a hearing loss: coping strategies. *Nurse Education*, **3 (4)**, 7–11

Burnfield, A. (1985) *Multiple Sclerosis: A Personal Exploration*, Souvenir Press, London

Campling, J. (1981) (ed.) *Images of Ourselves: Women with Disabilities Talking*, Routledge & Kegan Paul, London

Chartered Society of Physiotherapy (1984) *How to Become a Chartered Physiotherapist*, London

Chickadonz, G. H. (1983) Educating a deaf nursing student. *Nursing and Health Care*, **4 (6)**, 327–333

Chinnery, B. (1991) Equal opportunities for disabled people in the caring professions: window dressing or commitment? *Disability, Handicap and Society*, **6 (3)**, 253–258

Cole, A. (1987) Limited access. *Nursing Times*, **83 (24)**, 29–30

The College of Radiographers (1985) *Radiography—Your Career?*, London

Craik, C. (1990) Disability need not be a barrier to a career in occupational therapy. *Contact*, **66**, 14–16

Cumberbatch, G. and Negrine, R. (1992) *Images of Disability on Television*, Routledge, London

Darnbrough, A. and Kinrade, D. (1981) The disabled person and employment. In *Disability: Legislation and Practice*, (ed. D. Guthrie), Macmillan Press, London

Faulder, C. (1985) *Whose Body Is It?* Virago Press, London

Foucault, M. (1967) *Madness and Civilisation*, Tavistock Publications, London

French, S. (1986) Handicapped people in the health and caring professions—attitudes, practices and experiences. MSc dissertation, South Bank Polytechnic, London

French, S. (1987) Attitudes of physiotherapists to the recruitment of handicapped and disabled people into the physiotherapy profession. *Physiotherapy*, **73 (7)**, 363–367

French, S. (1988) Experiences of disabled health and caring professions. *Sociology of Health and Illness*, **10 (2)**, 170–188

French, S. (1990a) The advantages of visual impairment: some physiotherapists' views. *New Beacon*, **75 (872)**, 1–6

French, S. (1990b) Visually handicapped physiotherapists: are their educational needs being met? *Educare*, **37**, 12–19

French, S. (in progress) Doctoral research. South Bank University, London

Gavin, A. (1980) Meeting the challenge of professional social work: education of the hearing impaired. *American Annals of the Deaf*, December, **125**, 1086–1090

Goffman, I. (1968) *Stigma*, Penguin Books, Harmondsworth

Goffman, I. (1969) *The Presentation of Self in Everyday Life*, Penguin Books, Harmondsworth

Helman, C. (1984) *Culture, Health and Illness*, Butterworth-Heinemann, Oxford

Hughes, E. C. (1946) Institutions. In *New Outline of the Principles of Sociology* (ed. A. M. Lee), Barnes & Noble, New York

Hutchins, T. V. (1978) Affirmative action for the physically disabled in social work education. *Journal of Education for Social Work*, **14 (3)**, 64–70

Kettle, M. (1979) *Disabled People and Their Employment*, Association of Disabled Professionals, Banstead

Libman, G. (1983) Doctor who overcomes deafness. *Synapse*, **4 (5)**, 2–3

McKnight, J. (1981) Professionalised service and disabling help. In *Handicap in a Social World*, (eds A. Brechin, P. Liddiard and J. Swain), Hodder & Stoughton, Sevenoaks

Moon, P. (1990) *What Happens When Nurses Become Disabled?* The Royal Association for Disability and Rehabilitation, London

Morris, J. (1989) *Able Lives*, The Women's Press, London

O'Hare, C. and Thomson, D. (1991) Experiences of physiotherapists with physical disabilities. *Physiotherapy*, **77 (6)**, 374–377

Pearson, M. (1987) The great divide. *Nursing Times*, **83 (24)**, 25–26

Rieser, R. (1992a) Stereotypes of disabled people. In *Disability Equality in the Classroom: A Human Rights Issue*, (eds R. Rieser and M. Mason), Disability Equality in Education, London

Rieser, R. (1992b) Children's literature. In *Disability Equality in the Classroom: A Human Rights Issue*, (eds R. Rieser and M. Mason), Disability Equality in Education, London

Royal College of Nursing (1985) *Health Screening of Entrants to Nurse Training*, London

Safilios-Rothschild, C. (1976) Disabled person's self-definitions and their implications for rehabilitation. In *Rehabilitation: Supplementary Readings* (ed. V. Finkelstein), Open University Press, Milton Keynes

Scott, R. A. (1969) *The Making of Blind Men*, Russell Sage Foundation, New York

Scrivens, K. (1982) The National Health Service: origins and issues. In *Sociology as Applied to Medicine*, (eds G. L. Patrick and G. Scambler), Bailliere Tindall, London

Shearer, A. (1981) *Disability: Whose Handicap?* Basil Blackwell, Oxford

Smith, A. and Jacobson, B. (1988) *The Nation's Health*, King's Fund Publishing Office, London

Stetten, D. (1983) Tomorrow's physician. *Pharos*, **45 (3)**, 35–41

Sutherland, A. T. (1981) *Disabled We Stand*, Souvenir Press, London

Teager, D. P. G. (1987) The visually handicapped physiotherapist – the British experience. *International Disability Studies*, **8**, 134–143

Turner, C. (1984) Who cares? *Occupational Health*, **36 (10)**, 449–452

Wainapel, S. F. (1987) The physically disabled physician. *Journal of the American Medical Association*, **257 (21)**, 2936–2938

Wainapel, S. F. and Bernbaum, M. (1986) The physician with visual impairment and blindness. *Archives of Ophthalmology*, **104**, 498–502

Watkins, S. (1987) *Medicine and Labour*, Lawrence Wishart, London

Weller, L. and Grunes, S. (1988) Does contact with the mentally ill affect nurses' attitudes to mental illness? *British Journal of Medical Psychology*, **61**, 277–284

Young, G. (1981) A woman in medicine: reflections from the inside. In *Women, Health and Reproduction*, (ed. H. Roberts), Routledge & Kegan Paul, London

17

Disability and legislation

Ken Davis

For over four centuries in Britain, where disabled people have been among those singled out for legal treatment, we have been dealt with not as equal citizens with a right to full participation in the social mainstream, but as a problem in need of special treatment. Countless millions of pounds have been and are quite happily spent on research into why we are the way we are, on attempts to cure us, or rehabilitate us, or conductively educate us, or in some other way make us approximate to able-bodiedness, or make us fit into a society designed to serve and perpetuate able-bodied interests. And when despite all this effort we don't quite fit, or can't quite function, when we can't find jobs, millions more pounds are spent on social security, or welfare services, or heart-warming charitable endeavours designed to compensate in some way for the personal tragedy that has befallen us.

Over time, disabled people have moved from acquiescence, to uncertainty, discontent and, in recent years, to outright anger with this situation. We have been saying through our own organizations that our disability is caused not by the state of our bodies, but by the state of our society. We have said that we do not want legislation which treats us as people with special needs, but which instead outlaws and requires removal of the environmental and social barriers which prevent us from participating in the ordinary activities of daily life on equal terms. We have pointed out that we need legislation which enables us to take control of our lives, live independently and make a contribution to society. Until this kind of legislation has been enacted, we have warned that countless millions more pounds will be wasted just keeping us in a state of dependency and second-class citizenship.

In order to get this message across, campaigns have been launched, initiatives taken and efforts of many other kinds made, to try and bring to a halt this continued waste of public funds. Despite this, the vast majority of disabled people seeking work remain unemployed; millions exist on a State benefit system which is under attack; and we still find ourselves segregated, excluded and discriminated against in almost every aspect of social life. The disabled people's movement, through its national representative voice, the British Council of Organizations of Disabled People (BCODP), has been driven, as a result, to demand that the government takes action to bring an end to discrimination and secure for disabled people a proper legal foundation of equal citizenship. The remainder of this article considers some of the background events and issues, and reviews aspects of recent legislative activity which have moved disabled people into this position of political struggle.

Early paternalistic State provision

At first blush, it can seem hard to understand how it can be that, for all the improvements brought about in our lives by the Welfare State compared with the days of the Poor Law, disabled people are still unable to share equally in the society of which we are part. Yet it is our experience that most of the things it provides have never been asked for by disabled people, that they segregate us in a way which is a disgrace in any civilized society, that they make us dependent and unproductive, and often make us feel as though we should be eternally grateful for the beneficence of a caring State. It is plain enough that Poor Law paternalism has simply been replaced by a new era of welfare paternalism, as commentators like Oliver have pointed out:

> social policies, state provision and professional practice has failed disabled people ever since the welfare state began. . . . I suspect I won't be giving disabled people news that they didn't already know and won't have experienced for however long they have been disabled . . . the Welfare State has been based on paternalism at least since 1945 and if you don't think so, read the Beveridge Report, read the preamble to any of the legislation, the National Assistance Act and any of that stuff—it is paternalism. (Oliver, 1993: 13)

But then, on reflection, the Welfare State was far from revolutionary in its approach to dealing with the basic risks, requirements and contingencies of life. As with some of the earlier social welfare measures brought in at the time of Balfour and Lloyd George around the turn of the century, Baron Beveridge's grand plan sought to spike the guns of socialism by basing itself not on a scheme of free allowances from the State on the principle of 'from each according to his means, to each according to his needs', but by paying benefits as of right by virtue of contributions paid, on the insurance principle first established in the 1911 National Insurance Act. The new welfare arrangements very much emerged out of the incrementalist and paternalistic mould in which the character of British social policy development was set.

The National Assistance Act of 1948 referred to by Oliver starts with the somewhat over optimistic preamble that 'the existing Poor Law shall cease to have effect and shall be replaced' (Fraser, 1984: 229). However, it perpetuated the hated means test; continued the dumping of disabled people in institutions; in line with the 43rd Act of Elizabeth in 1602 (the Old Poor Law) required inmates to be charged (Fisher and Jurica, 1977) with the cost of being isolated and segregated from the social mainstream; and fostered the use of segregated services like workshops and hostels run by the charitable voluntary organizations for disabled people which, since the middle of the nineteenth century, have become a powerful vested interest in disability services.

This is not to suggest that the idea of welfare is wrong nor that it does not bring undoubted benefits for its beneficiaries. But we should be keenly critical of the form it takes in our own lives, and our demand today for welfare which supports our independence, social integration and equal citizenship is an expression of that duty. Yet we can understand that in the feudal Britain of the fourteenth century, say, when the earliest seeds of future disability legislation were being sown in the precursive legislation to the Old Poor Law, it would have been a very different matter. Early poor relief, like later welfare measures, came out of a fear by the ruling class of social unrest. It was a product of its own time. To be sure, successive generations of poor law officials, welfare administrators and caring professionals have turned it to their own advantage. Now we must ensure that the State maintains the collective commitment to fund welfare provision, but that it is used to secure our full participation and equality.

In this sense, we can see that early disabled people's groups (Pagel, 1988) like the British Deaf Association (1890) and the National League of the Blind (1899), which adopted an approach to welfare which was to last at least until the 1970s, were responding appropriately to the harsh circumstances facing their members around the turn of the century. In the context of a growing labour movement and emerging social welfare arrangements, they were taking up a progressive position. The League campaigned hard (NLB, 1988) for the 1920 and 1938 Blind Persons Acts, which brought some advances for visually-impaired people. But these groups, as with the Disablement Income Group (DIG) some forty years later, were less interested in the underlying reasons as to why welfare was needed than in improving the immediate circumstances of their lives, and gaining for themselves some equivalence with non-disabled contemporaries. (For further discussion of the disability movement, the reader is referred to chapter 6.)

Later legislation—a denial of our rights

In order to bring about the kind of legislation needed to break the mould of paternalistic State provision, disabled people first had to break the mould in which our own expectations were set. We needed to overturn the power of the medical model and what Oliver (1990: 1) has described as the personal tragedy theory of disability which underpinned welfare benefits and services. Among the ways this change came about were our own struggles to change institutional regimes (Hunt, 1992: 30) or escape them (Davis, 1993); developments in integrated and independent living abroad; the unfulfilled promises of the Chronically Sick and Disabled Persons Act (CSDPA) of 1973; and the failure of DIG's campaign for a national disability income.

Once the Union of the Physically Impaired against Segregation, set up in 1974 to spearhead a collective struggle for change, had defined disability as being socially caused, the way had been paved for a civil rights campaign to outlaw discrimination. It has been suggested that this:

> signalled the end of the welfare oriented 'begging bowl' period, and with it the idea that the 'experts' could administer away disabled people's problems for them. This made the early Seventies the pivotal period in the development of the movement. From this point on, the emphasis was to be less on appeals to able-bodied people's better nature, polite petitions or orderly marches on Parliament Square, but more on the mobilisation of a democratically organised, politically aware movement. (Davis, 1993: 288)

In the face of a more critical approach to disability issues which followed the formation of the Union, the CSDPA, hyped up as being the start of a new era for disabled people, was shown to amount to little more than a repetition of the well-worn parliamentary device to stifle the growing demands for more substantial social change. It had been deliberately weakened when the bill was in committee stage, a process noticeably applied in sections which might enable disabled people to participate in the social mainstream: housing, public buildings and facilities and so on. As a result, its main focus is not on socially caused disability, but on individuals and their presumed welfare needs. The state of mind of the drafters of this legislation can be judged from the kind of welfare needs that can be met under section 2 of the Act, which includes things like telephones, wireless and television, educational and library facilities, lectures, games, holidays and outings.

Even the 1990 NHS and Community Care Act, accompanied as it has been by a welter of politic rhetoric about independence, choice and control, and backed by the government's touching belief in the power of market forces to produce it, has failed to break the chains which bind us into unnecessary dependence. It gives disabled people no rights, and indeed has supplanted what limited rights to representation and assessment for services could have been available to us, had the government chosen to implement the relevant sections of the 1986 Disabled Persons (Services, Consultation and Representation) Act.

Indeed an important adjunct to community care in the shape of an Independent Living Fund, which placed payments directly in the hands of disabled people in order to purchase, under their own control, personal assistance for independent living, has been supplanted in 1993 with a new fund which restores the binding link to and dependence on professionally provided social services. To underpin and secure this preservation of professional power and control, the government has consistently refused to introduce legislation which would make it legal for local authorities themselves to make direct payments which would put some purchasing power, choice and control back into disabled people's own hands. The Derbyshire Coalition of Disabled People, commenting on the implementation of community care in the editorial column of a recent newsletter said:

> Instead of giving us rights, the Community Care Act puts us in the Limboland of uncertainty between a mixed market place of providers on the one hand, and professional controllers of services on the other. Never has there been such a need for a completely new approach to welfare: the kind of welfare which is based on individual, enforcable rights and entitlements. The right wing view of the market place as the source of meeting our needs is as hopeless and redundant as the hope that they will somehow be met through the state controlled system of democratic accountability—which in practice is accountable not to us, but the infinitely more powerful interest groups which feed on our artificially created dependency. (DCDP, 1993)

This call for a new approach to the idea and practice of welfare echoes many of the arguments which were being developed twenty years earlier by the Union of the Physically Impaired. In those days, UPIAS held firmly to the view that the proper way forward for disabled people was through a 'serious struggle for the right to paid, integrated employment and full participation in the mainstream of life' (UPIAS, 1976: 15). This view has gradually come to be adopted more widely as the disabled people's movement has grown and now finds expression through the campaign led by BCODP (Barnes, 1991) for anti discrimination legislation (ADL), referred to in the opening paragraphs of this chapter.

The fight for anti-discrimination legislation

The first steps towards putting ADL on any parliamentary agenda, however, were taken not by UPIAS but by the Committee on Restrictions against Disabled People (CORAD) under the chairmanship of Peter Large. Set up in the final days of the Labour administration in January 1979 as a way of furthering the work of the Silver Jubilee Access Committee (SJAC), CORAD was charged with the task of considering 'the architectural and social barriers which may result in discrimination against disabled people and prevent them making full use of facilities available to the general public; and to make recommendations' (Large, 1982: 1). The first of the Report's 42 recommendations was that 'there should be legislation to make discrimination on the grounds of disability illegal' (Large, 1982: 53) and that it should cover such instances wherever they might occur, but particularly in the areas of employment, education, transport and the provision of goods, facilities and services. When CORAD began its work, there was a good deal of optimism that its findings would find their way on to the statute book since the committee had been set up by Alf Morris, the Labour MP now seeking parliamentary support for his Civil Rights Bill. However, the elections of May 1979 and the arrival of a Conservative government completely altered the climate of political support.

By the time the CORAD report had been produced, in 1982, and despite the arousal of a heightened sense of public awareness to some extent generated by the designation of 1981 as an International Year of Disabled People, the chances of any anti-discrimination bill finding a majority in parliament had almost completely disappeared. Several attempts to introduce such legislation in one form or another failed repeatedly throughout the 1980s. Barnes (1991: 235–6) notes nine such tries between 6 July 1982, when Jack Ashley MP introduced the Disablement (Prohibition of Unjustifiable Discrimination) Bill and the presentation of John Hughes' Disability Discrimination Bill on 6 February 1991.

Elsewhere in the world, however, the situation has been more hopeful and positive. The Canadian government took steps to give some constitutional protection to disabled citizens in 1983 and in 1990, after long campaigning by disabled people and their supporters in the United States, the much more comprehensive Americans with Disabilities Act (ADA) came into being. Justin Dart, one of the disabled campaigners who worked on the ADA, echoed the same economic basis of argument which was the basis of the UPIAS case for change in Britain during the 1970s, as part of the pressure which was brought to bear on the Bush administration of the time. Just before the ADA

Bill was passed by Congress, he said that the economic cost of segregating millions of disabled people from the productive mainstream of American life was running at $300 billion per year and failure to enact ADA:

> would lead directly to more unemployment and increasing dependency on massive, paternalistic welfare systems. It would guarantee higher taxes, higher government, business and family budgets, and higher public deficits. An effective ADA will free millions of people with disabilities from the bondage of dependency, enabling them to become employees, taxpayers and customers. It will save billions for government and directly profit every business and every citizen. (Dart, 1990)

Congress finally passed the bill into law on 26 July 1990, acknowledging in the preamble that some 43 million disabled Americans had historically suffered and continued to suffer isolation, segregation and discrimination in critical areas such as employment, housing, public buildings, education, transportation, communication, recreation, health services, voting and access to public services. As with the BCODP case for ADL here in Britain, they accepted the depth of institutional and various other forms of discrimination:

> including outright intentional exclusion, the discriminatory effects of architectural, transportation, and communication barriers, overprotective rules and policies, failure to make modifications to existing facilities and practices, exclusionary qualification standards and criteria, segregation, and relegation to lesser services, programs, activities, benefits, jobs, or other opportunities. (ADA, 1990).

Congress concluded that the cost to the United States involved billions of dollars in unnecessary expenses resulting from dependency and non-productivity. The continued existence of unfair and unnecessary discrimination and prejudice was thus intolerable, and they agreed that the nation's proper goals would be to assure equality of opportunity, full participation, independent living and economic self-sufficiency for disabled people in American society.

In Australia, the Disability Discrimination Act 1992 received the Royal Assent on 5 November 1992 with the object of eliminating, as far as possible, discrimination against persons on the ground of disability in the areas of:

> (a) (i) work, accommodation, education, access to premises, clubs and sport; and (ii) the provision of goods, facilities, services and land; and (iii) existing laws; and (iv) the administration of Commonwealth laws and programs; and (b) to ensure, as far as practicable, that persons with disabilities have the same rights to equality before the law as the rest of the community; and (c) to promote recognition and acceptance within the community of the principle that persons with disabilities have the same fundamental rights as the rest of the community. (DDA, 1992)

In New Zealand, the Human Rights Act 1994, which is designed to consolidate and amend earlier race relations and human rights legislation and give better protection for minority rights in New Zealand in line with United Nations declarations extensively includes disabled people among its provisions. The Human Rights Act (1994) seeks to make discrimination against disabled people unlawful in relation to access to public places, vehicles and facilities, in the provision of goods and services and in a variety of other circumstances and situations. In each of these anti-discrimination enactments, unlawful discrimination in employment matters takes a prominent place, indicating that the adverse economic aspect of socially caused disability (discrimination) is a feature, the undesirability of which has finally dawned in the consciousness of the governments concerned.

The extent to which this was understood in the United States is indicated by Dick Thornburgh (1990), then US Attorney General, in a speech to the Eighth Annual Government Conference on the Employment of Persons with Disabilities. Referring to the widespread job discrimination in the private sector which had left 58 per cent of disabled men and 80 per cent of disabled women jobless, he picked up on the question of comparative cost, ie the cost of passing or not passing the ADA. He said that, for example, widening a door to permit wheelchair access could cost as much as $300 to $600 per door, but it was also known that the widening must be done, not only because it is right:

> but because it is in truth, the only cost effective solution to a dependency that costs our society well over $100 billion a year. Only through empowering this first generation and all coming generations as productive citizens can we overcome this defeating equation. Dependency equals a $45,000 annual cost to maintain each unemployed person with a disability or $2 million over an unwillingly dependent and idle lifetime. (Thornburgh, 1990)

Nevertheless, the effect of pressure and lobbying by groups with a vested interest in stopping or neutralizing the effect of ADL can be seen in the variety of conditions, exceptions and delaying devices built into the US as well as the Australian and New Zealand legislation, echoing the resistance to earlier civil rights measures. Justin Dart (1990) noted in the United States that powerful vested interests were pushing for 'separate but equal' facilities and other discriminatory barriers which would perpetuate the unemployment, impoverishment and welfare dependency of disabled people, but went on to argue on the eve of the passage of the Americans with Disabilities Act that:

> This landmark legislation—a world first—provides citizens with disabilities the same 'clear mandate for the elimination of discrimination'

> which other minorities attained more than two decades ago . . . (yet) . . . professional lobbyists are flooding Congressional offices and the public media with strident claims that ADA would force backbreaking costs and lawsuits on business. These claims are groundless. They reflect the same obsolete attitudes, unfounded fears and erroneous doomsday predictions that have greeted all previous extensions of basic civil rights protections. (Dart, 1990)

The extent to which deployment of the economic argument and link with other civil rights legislation might budge the British government is hard to judge. On the latter, there has been no matter of principle or precedent in the way since the passage of race relations and sex discrimination legislation in the 1960s and 1970s. So far, the present Minister for the Disabled has used attempts to make comparisons between ADL and legislation to combat discrimination on grounds of race and gender as an opportunity to try and undermine unity across the movement. He has tried to argue that, unlike women and black people, disabled people are not an homogenous group and people with different kinds of disability experience different kinds of discrimination and thus, (almost as though he were unaware of ADL elsewhere in the world) it would be too complicated to legislate.

Since the failure of John Hughes' Disability Discrimination Bill in 1991 and the 'talking out' of Alf Morris' Civil Rights (Disabled Persons) Bill early in 1992, when the latter was re-introduced in February 1993, Morris himself deployed the economic case by referring in the Commons to the gains in terms of national economic wealth to be made by the integration of disabled people into mainstream social life:

> enacting civil rights legislation . . . adds to wealth by reducing their dependence on benefits and increasing the contribution they can make. This is no academic point. When the Americans with Disabilities Act was passed through Congress, the realisation of that effect secured the support of more and more of its former critics. They began to talk more not only of its possible cost, but also of its undoubted economic and social value. (Hansard, 1993: 1142)

However, to date, no amount of polite argument has been able to change the Conservative government's position on ADL. The government's chosen course is well articulated by its minister, whose task is to manage public pressure and protect the government's broader policy of cutting public expenditure and having individuals provide for themselves. The management of pressure from the disability lobby is achieved by way of pointing to what successes can be discovered resulting from their 'education and persuasion' and 'sector by sector' approach, coupled with casting doubts on the effectiveness of overarching ADL where 'the costs are unquantifiable and which is likely to lead to excessive bureaucracy and a beanfeast for the legal profession' and where it 'would imply considerable costs for employers, suppliers and the Government' (Hansard, 1993: 1178, 1185).

Conclusion

As this article is being prepared for publication in the opening weeks of 1994, so the disabled people's movement in Britain is preparing itself to campaign behind what is turning into an almost ritual like re-introduction of the Civil Rights Bill in the spring. Echoing many other struggles in the past, from attempts to abolish slavery to efforts to extend the franchise to women, on eleven occasions throughout the lifetime of the present Conservative government, legal protection for disabled people against discrimination has been sought from parliament and denied. Whilst the repeated presentation of the arguments has made some impression on the present minister, who now says that no one can 'doubt for a moment that there continues to be considerable discrimination against disabled people', nevertheless 'his head and his heart divide' (Hansard, 1993: 1175) about legislating to prevent the daily degrading process happening in the lives of six million people across the length and breadth of Britain.

On the back of this kind of suffocating complacency, Britain is rapidly becoming one of the more backward nations in the Commonwealth, as others have moved to take legislative action. Given the traditional attachment of the average Tory to the monarchy, and despite the fortunate fact that it is now more like the stamp of a visa than the threat of a veto, it is ironic that the obduracy of the Conservative government has put the Queen in the position of being able to give the Royal Assent to laws which protect disabled people from discrimination in the farthest flung comers of the Commonwealth, whilst being unable to offer the same protection to us here on her own doorstep. Quite clearly, those in power feel they can brush our interests aside with impunity.

Nevertheless there is a build up of pressure on the government, as well as on the so-called caring professionals, their unions and professional associations whose well-paid careers have often been constructed on the backs of our segregation and artificially created dependency. As this pressure grows, we can expect the former to try and hold the established policy line with a pre-emptive legislative strike designed to avoid more radical measures, and the latter to continue to divide into two camps: one overtly in support of our movement and its demands, and the other covertly against—but with a substantial number in both with a tactical eye on retaining as much power and control over our lives as they can hang on to. But as always, the ultimate outcome will depend on ourselves.

References

Americans with Disabilities Act (ADA) (1990) Public Law 101–336, 104 Stat. 327, US Congress

Barnes, C. (1991) *Disabled People in Britain and Discrimination: A Case for Anti-Discrimination Legislation*, Hurst & Co., London, in association with The British Council of Organizations of Disabled People, Belper, Derbyshire

Dart, J. (1990), Editorial. *Congressional Task Force on the Rights and Empowerment of Americans with Disabilities*, Library 7, Rights and Legislation, Disabilities Forum, Compuserve

Davis, K. (1993) On the movement. In *Disabling Barriers—Enabling Environments*, (eds J. Swain, V. Finkelstein, S. French and M. Oliver), Sage, London

Davis, M. (1993) Personal Assistance – Notes on the historical context in making our own choices (ed. C. Barnes). British Council of Organizations of Disabled People, Belper, Derbyshire

Disability Discrimination Act (DDA) (1992) No. 135 of 1992, The Parliament of Australia

Derbyshire Coalition of Disabled People (DCDP) (1993) Editorial. *INFO*, 10, DCDP, Clay Cross, Derbyshire

Fisher, H. E. S. and Jurica, A. R. J., (eds) (1977), 14 Elizabeth, c. 5, Statutes of the Realm, IV, Part I. In *Documents in English Economic History: England from 1000 to 1760*, G Bell & Sons Ltd, London

Fraser, D., (1984), *The Evolution of the British Welfare State*, Macmillan, London

Hansard, (1993), *Parliamentary Debates*, 26 February, HMSO, London

Human Rights Act (1994) 1993, No. 82, Parliament of New Zealand

Hunt, J. (1992) The disabled people's movement between 1960–1986 and its effect upon the development of community support services. Unpublished MA dissertation, The Polytechnic of East London

Large, P. (1982) *Report by the Committee on Restrictions against Disabled People*, HMSO, London

National League of the Blind and Disabled (1988) A brief history of the national league of the blind and disabled 1899–1987, *Year Book 1988*, NLBD, Manchester

Oliver, M. (1990) *The Politics of Disablement*, Macmillan, London

Oliver, M. (1993) Moving on: from welfare paternalism to welfare citizenship. In *INFO* 10, Derbyshire Coalition of Disabled People, Clay Cross, Derbyshire

Pagel, M. (1988), On Our Own Behalf—An Introduction to the Self-Organisation of Disabled People, Greater Manchester Coalition of Disabled People, Manchester

Thornburgh, D. (1990) The promise of the Americans with Disabilities Act. Speech at the Office of Personnel Management Eighth Annual Governmentwide Conference on the Employment of Persons with Disabilities, Library 7, Rights and Legislation, Disabilities Forum, Compuserve

Union of the Physically Impaired against Segregation (UPIAS) (1976) *Fundamental Principles of Disability*, London, UPIAS

18

Innovative practice

Louise Silburn, Devala Dookun and Chris Jones

In this chapter three examples of innovative practice by health and welfare professionals will be explained. The first account, by Louise Silburn, examines how a team of therapists worked with severely disabled people within the philosophy of the social model of disability. The second account, by Devala Dookun, explains a family and child-centred approach to the treatment of disabled children. The third account, by Chris Jones, explains how a multidisciplinary team of professionals assisted multiply disabled people to find employment.

A social model in a medical world: the development of the integrated living team as part of the strategy for younger physically disabled people in North Derbyshire

A young disabled unit: to be or not to be?

In 1985 North Derbyshire Health Authority started planning how to spend the £430,000 they had been given for services to younger disabled people. They assumed that they would do what most of their neighbouring authorities had done and build a Younger Disabled Unit (YDU). A newly formed joint planning group, including representatives of the Derbyshire Coalition of Disabled People and the Derbyshire Centre for Integrated Living (DCIL), were asked to discuss the issues.

Senior nurses and the district medical officer felt very strongly that a small YDU was needed in North Derbyshire. The Coalition and DCIL put forward equally strongly the view that putting money into such a unit kept vital resources away from the community services that disabled people needed in order to stay out of such units. The ideas, language and experience of the two groups, and the early stages of planning, were fraught with conflict.

Disabled people's needs and priorities: a survey

The short-term planning solution was to commission a survey which would establish what the expressed needs of disabled people in North Derbyshire were. The research was carried out by the University of Nottingham (Silburn, 1988) and was based on seven needs as defined by disabled people in Derbyshire, as well as planning issues facing health and social services. The seven needs were for: information, technical aids, housing, counselling, transport, personal assistance and access. Particular services, such as physiotherapy, chiropody, drugs, day services and domiciliary services were also scrutinized.

What the survey showed was that disabled people wanted community services; they wanted information and more broadly-based services, in areas such as peer counselling, rather than specific professional interventions. The survey results strongly indicated the interlinking nature of the seven needs and the necessity to plan services in an integrated way. The planning group began to plan community services to reflect the needs as perceived by its population of disabled people. This emphasis was very unusual and highly challenging to health professionals who were used to being in control of decisions of this nature. Eventually a community strategy was agreed, with a proportion of the available finances being set aside for an integrated living co-ordinator and a flexible budget.

The integrated living team: planning and philosophy

The role of the integrated living co-ordinator was to manage the budget which would help people to move out of hospital quickly, and stop them being admitted inappropriately. The planning group also decided to use some of the money to pay for an occupational therapist, a speech therapist and a physiotherapist who, working in a team, would be managed by the integrated living co-ordinator. I was appointed to the post of co-ordinator with a background of work as joint director of the Derbyshire Centre of Integrated Living. My knowledge and experience of planning and providing services for disabled people came from the disability movement. As a result of this appointment, therefore, the health service was endorsing the creation of a team whose philosophy and practice were firmly rooted in the social model of disability.

The role of the integrated living team member

It is accepted by all team members that the people with whom we work have requirements which need to be fulfilled as quickly as possible and in a way which gives them control over the process of achieving integrated living. It is therefore necessary to adopt a key-worker approach whereby one team member is responsible for working with each disabled person on all aspects of his or her move out of hospital, or on helping the person remain in the community if there is a risk of inappropriate hospital admission. The therapists use each other's professional expertise in discussion and advice and from time to time conduct joint visits if specialist assessments are needed. As the team members have grown in confidence and commitment to this new way of working, they have tried to drop any reference to their original professional titles. This practice has caused uncomfortable feelings among health service staff in other areas whose habitual first question to the team members and myself is 'What are you?'

The bulk of the work of the team revolves around the seven needs which are used as the basis of service planning. The disabled people with whom the team works may have health needs which are being met by hospitals or primary health-care services, but the reason they need help from the team is because they do not have access to the appropriate non-medical services they require to live comfortable and secure lives in the community.

When a team member visits someone for the first time, he or she assesses the services required by reference to the seven needs, only the most basic and immediately relevant details about medical and personal factors are used in the initial assessment. The service the team provides does not have to conform to the procedures laid down by a department or by the boundaries imposed by a professional qualification; it has been developed to be specifically useful to disabled people in particular circumstances.

Criteria for referral to the team

The team work with people aged between 16 and 64 who are severely physically impaired and who find themselves in the following circumstances: in hospital and needing to move out into the community; at risk of inappropriate hospital admission. 'Inappropriate' means, in this context, that the person is not ill and is not in need of medical attention in hospital. Another way of defining our criteria is to say that the person would have been admitted to a YDU had there been one in the district.

The flexible budget

The budget is the key to creative working by the team members. It allows them to discuss different options with the disabled people with whom they work, and allows them to have access to the funds necessary to finance the disabled people's choices. It is mainly used for non-recurrent expenditure, such as technical aids which are not available from other services, adaptations, personal assistance in the home, transport and holidays. However, it can be used for anything thought appropriate to help someone remain in the community or to enable someone to move out of hospital.

It is often used in conjunction with other resources or funding to make the best use of the available money. It can therefore be used to top up disabled facilities grants, and to make major adaptations a reality for people for whom means testing would otherwise make changes to their homes impossible. It can be used to pay for personal assistance in someone's home for an interim period until social services have recruited staff to continue with the long-term commitment. It has also been used as a successful stop-gap while people have awaited Independent Living Fund money.

Examples of work

The team's work with disabled people can be broken down into five categories:

1. Some people are admitted to hospital following an accident or illness that results in physical impairment. They will require varying degrees of medical treatment before they go home and may be referred to a specialist in-patient rehabilitation facility such as a spinal or head injury unit.

   People in this group often require substantial adaptations to their homes before they can return to them, or their family circumstances may change so that returning to their original homes may no longer be an option. They may therefore remain in hospital wards although they are no longer in need of medical care.

   Most of the people we have helped to move out of hospital have gone home fairly quickly and services have gradually been developed around them. For some this is not possible; this may be because they are homeless, or because their home is unsuitable even for temporary occupation. For these people we have embarked upon complex joint projects with council housing departments and environmental health departments, drawing up plans with the disabled person, his or her family, and the health authority works department. The process for some people is frustrating and slow, despite our budget and time. Yet involvement in the process has been helpful to people adjusting to a changed body, a new lifestyle and new challenges.

2. Another group of people with whom the team works are those who are in hospital because they have been inappropriately admitted; for example, they may have been admitted to be 'sorted out'. 'Sorting out' means that their drugs are reviewed, the hospital occupational therapist and physiotherapist work with them, and they have a rest in hospital while their carers rest at home.

   As a result of this stay in hospital it often become evident that the root of the problem is a lack of accessible housing, poor technical aids and not enough support for either the disabled person or the carer in the form of practical help or emotional/social release. In this situation the social worker contacts the integrated living team who then starts to 'sort out' the social environment which is disabling that person.

3. For some people with degenerative, terminal diseases, such as motor neurone disease (MND), a joint approach to services has been developed. The hospice in Chesterfield will take people with MND into their day hospital, and then later for respite care and the final stages of illness. The integrated living team can work with people from diagnosis of MND onwards, to ensure that they stay at home as long as possible, anticipating communication needs, personal assistance requirements and planning any adaptations that may be necessary.

4. Working with people who are at risk of inappropriate hospital admission accounts for over half of the team's work. A disabled person can be inappropriately admitted because of the illness of a carer or the possibility of a carer leaving altogether. Another reason could be a deterioration in the person's physical state which is not matched by an increase in support at home. Sometimes the cause is relationship or emotional problems that have come to a head.

   When first visiting someone at home the team member will have some idea about what is threatening to make his or her admission to hospital likely, but working through the seven needs with people will reveal a much broader picture of their lives. If the primary requirement is the relief of stress the team will often organize a holiday, to be taken fairly quickly, and then spend longer looking at personal assistance, counselling, technical aids and housing issues which might have caused the stress in the first place.

5. The final group of people consists of those for whom ill health is the result of social problems. For most people, such ill health would not warrant admission to hospital. For disabled people it

often does because it is the emergency response forced on the GPs who are given neither the role nor the resources to tackle the root cause. Also, for disabled people, ill health can lead to complaints that are more serious and difficult to treat.

The team has successfully worked with people who were frequently being admitted to hospital so that they can stay in the community in better health as a result of better organized and higher-quality services.

The way forward: rehabilitation or integrated living?

The integrated living team is operating at the interface of social and medical models of care. The medical model is enshrined in the rehabilitation service, which still dominates the health service's view of what disabled people need. The concept of the disabling society is not one which is seriously considered when delivering health services to disabled people.

Yet it is questionable to what extent disabled people would want to be rehabilitated if they lived in a world where the struggle to learn to walk a few yards on crutches was made pointless by decent wheelchairs and a barrier-free environment. The work of the integrated living team is based firmly in the realm of creating for disabled people as barrier-free an environment, in the widest sense, as possible, to enable them to live secure and integrated lives. Therefore rehabilitation is not practised by the team and this is what makes it so threatening to health professionals rooted in the rehabilitation tradition.

The medical rehabilitation world can be a comfortable place and some of its most powerful exponents can treat those of us living outside it with barely disguised contempt. It is sometimes hard for all of us in the team to resist the temptation to be part of that world by seeing disabled people's bodies as the problem and denying the disabling society. Yet in Derbyshire we work closely with disabled people for whom the disabling society is a reality, and through them derive support for our belief that working within a social model of disability is the most helpful service we can offer.

References

Silburn, L. (1988) *Disabled People: Their Needs and Priorities*, Benefits Research Unit, Department of Social Policy and Administration, University of Nottingham

(This is an edited version of a chapter which was originally published in *Disabling Barriers—Enabling Environments*, (eds J. Swain, V. Finkelstein, S. French and M. Oliver) (1993), Sage, London)

Individualized family service plans

(On behalf of the staff of the Child Development Centre, St George's Hospital, London.)

The team at the Child Development Centre at St George's Hospital, London, is gradually putting into action Individualized Family Service Plans (IFSP). The superintendent paediatric physiotherapist on the team was introduced to this approach at a symposium on family-centred intervention in the United States and this was reinforced when three of us working in the Child Development Centre, and a senior portage worker from the local education authority, attended a course at the Tavistock centre run by Naomi Dale entitled 'Working in Partnership with Families with Children with Long Term Special Needs'.

The underlying philosophy of IFSP is that 'families and professionals work together as a team to identify and mobilize formal and informal resources to help families reach their chosen goals,' (McGonigel et al., 1991: 1). This requires a considerable cultural shift on the part of professionals from their traditional role as the 'experts', who make decisions about what is best for the child and the family, to a more consumer-based model where they enable and empower the child and the family to make their own decisions regarding both needs and priorities. With IFSP a 'case manager' is initially identified by the professionals working with the family, but later it is hoped that the family will become its own case manager, or will select the person it would like to fulfil this role.

A fundamental aim of IFSP is to discover what the family's agenda is. This allows for the realistic setting of goals, and negotiation where necessary on what individuals (including family members) can and cannot provide. An additional and important function of IFSP is that it helps to identify areas of service delivery that need to be developed, or where a break in therapy may be indicated. We feel that this process encourages an open and honest atmosphere where both families and professionals are able to work and move forward together; on some occasions we agree to disagree.

Devising an individual family service plan

The process of arriving at an individualized family service plan involves the following stages:

1. The family are made aware of IFSP and how they can contribute to it. It is at this early stage that information, for example, booklets about local services, is provided.
2. The case manager arranges to meet the family at a time and in a place that is convenient for the family, for example at home in the evening so that a working parent can attend.
3. An interview takes place which is exploratory and relatively unstructured. The family and/or the child are facilitated and supported in identifying their main concerns and priorities. Part of the interview is spent in asking the family to describe their child in a few sentences and, if the child is able, he or she is encouraged to do the same. They are also asked to identify the important people in the family; in this context the word 'family' is used very loosely to include neighbours and friends who play a significant role.
4. The family then makes a list of three to five goals they would like to address over an agreed period of time, for example six months; this is done with reference to the priorities which they previously established. Their list of goals provides the basis for an action plan, where it is decided who will undertake the various tasks, and a time frame for the achievement of the goals. An important part of the plan is to identify what the child and family can do. The aim of IFSP is to empower the family and the child to value their existing strengths and networks of support (friends, churches, etc) rather than necessarily replacing them with professional systems and networks. Families are also encouraged to communicate with professionals directly, rather than through the case manager; considerable help and support may be needed to enable them to do all this effectively.
5. A date is agreed to review and update the plan. This date can of course, be deferred or brought forward if necessary.
6. A written copy of the plan is left with the family to consider for a day or two and, if they feel happy with it, the parents and/or child, as well as the case manager, sign it.

This way of working invites families and children to identify what *they* want rather than what we feel is right for them. This is challenging and certainly made us all review our practice; were we really providing the services disabled children and their families wanted, or were we merely doing what we felt comfortable with because 'that is what we'd always done'? We recognized our need for training, so time was set aside for sessions to build on previous knowledge and experience and to develop goal setting and interviewing skills. Initially we were concerned about dealing with requests which might go beyond our remit, or coping with interviews which veered off track, but through several long discussions these worries were allayed.

Giving information

It is recognized that families cannot make informed decisions unless they know what services and facilities are available (Cunningham and Davis, 1988). We were aware that as professionals we were often the 'gatekeepers' of knowledge, imparting small 'packages' of information according to our own perceptions and ideas of what a family needs. With this in mind we set about gathering comprehensive information to give to families, the challenge was to provide an extensive resource which was, at the same time, easy to use. We assembled the information into an A5 loose-leaf file where pages could be added, updated or removed, and where information pertaining to particular conditions could be inserted as appropriate. So far we have produced a prototype, making use of coloured papers to break the material into sections and graphics to reinforce important points and break up the text.

We have used IFSP, and the information file, with a small pilot group of families which is closely representative of those with whom we work, The response of this small group has been very positive; comments have included 'It's really started us thinking', 'it makes us realize we often set too many goals', 'it was really good to have someone who really listened to what I wanted', and, when speaking of the information file, 'although a lot to take on board, it's good to have it to refer to.'

Conclusion

Family led services and partnership is the cornerstone of our work, and with this end in view IFSP has been adopted. Individualized family service plans also provide a useful tool for measuring the outcomes of our work which, in turn, can be used for the purposes of auditing and quality assurance. We believe that the IFSP model of working will enable families to identify their own needs and the services they want, which in turn will enable us to identify priorities both in terms of current services and future developments.

References

Cunningham, C. and Davis, H. (1988) *Working with Parents: Frameworks for Collaboration*, Open University Press, Milton Keynes
McGonigel, M. J., Kaufman, B. K. and Johnson, B. H. (1991) *Guidelines and Recommended Practices for the Individualized Family Service Plan*, NEC*TAS (National Early Childhood Technical System) and ACCH (Association for the Care of Children's Health), USA

Further reading

Mitchell, D. and Brown, R. T. (eds) (1991) *Early Intervention Studies for Young Children with Special Needs*, Chapman & Hall, London
Meisels, S. J. and Shonkoff, J. P. (eds) (1990) *Handbook of Early Intervention*, Cambridge University Press, Cambridge

Acknowledgements

Thanks are extended to Chris Bungay, Superintendent Physiotherapist.

Employment for people with multiple disability

Increasingly society has come to recognize the damaging consequences of labelling disabled people and the dehumanizing effect of life in institutions (Ryan and Thomas, 1987; Potts and Fido, 1991). New services are being developed to reinstate the basic human rights of disabled people; supported employment services are currently the best example of an attempt to restore the right to work for people with a learning disability.

The rapid increase in supported employment services in recent years has highlighted a real commitment by some employers to include people with learning disabilities in the workplace (O'Brien, 1990), and has shown that people with learning disabilities are capable of holding down real jobs with the right support. In 1992 there were 1619 people who were ineligible for inclusion in unemployment statistics who were, nonetheless, being supported in jobs (National Development Team, 1992).

While most supported employment services are committed in principle to offering support to individuals regardless of their level of disability, in reality this does not happen. Only 1 per cent of people in supported employment have 'profound disabilities', and only 1 per cent come from 'special needs' or 'special care' units (National Development Team, 1992). Instead individuals with the most severe disabilities tend to be trapped in segregated settings undergoing therapeutic and educational programmes from which they can never graduate (Baumgart et al., 1982).

A project recently undertaken on Merseyside aimed to go some way towards rectifying this situation by increasing the number of people with multiple disability in work settings, using the supported employment model. For the purpose of the project a person with a multiple disability was defined as someone with a severe learning disability who had an additional physical disability and/or sensory disability and/or communication difficulty. Supported employment was defined by the National Development Team as 'real work in an integrated work setting with on-going support provided by a social services agency' (1992: 2).

The project team comprised a social worker, a clinical psychologist and an occupational therapist. The team's task was to develop expertise within a number of agencies so that they could offer a supported employment service to their clients with complex needs. The project was made possible by a change in the funding arrangements of services for people with learning disability. As people were moved out of local institutions money became available to provide good quality services to individuals.

There are many reasons why a person might choose to work and there are many benefits to be gained. These include an increase in status, developing self-identity, making new relationships, achieving financial security and gaining control over one's own life. Brown et al. (1984) suggest a hierarchy of priorities which service providers should consider when seeking employment on behalf of a severely disabled person. The highest priority should be to place the person in a non-segregated environment that offers access to meaningful work and an enhanced quality of life. Once placed in an enhancing environment efforts should be made to develop the individual's work skills and productivity. Finally, pay at the going rate should be negotiated.

Following these guidelines, the Merseyside project used O'Brien's 'framework for accomplishment' (1987) to ensure the person's quality of life was enhanced, employed 'systematic instruction' (Gold, 1980) to develop the individual's work skills, and made the work site and tasks accessible using individualized adaptations (Baumgart et al., 1982). Remuneration was always sought for work undertaken once an agreed level of productivity was reached.

The process used by the Merseyside project to obtain employment for people with multiple disability had four stages:

Stage 1   Information gathering and developing work notions
Stage 2   Job development
Stage 3   Job training and support
Stage 4   Evaluation

Stage 1: Information gathering and developing job notions

Before a work placement was sought information relating to the person's strengths, aptitudes, personal preferences, present lifestyle and desired lifestyle were gathered by the identified job trainer using a system resembling the 'getting to know you' process developed by Brost and Johnson (1982). This period also ensured that the individual and the job trainer felt comfortable together before entering the work-place. This was particularly important when assistance with personal care was needed before entering the workplace. The information was then brought to a 'job notion' meeting and was discussed under four headings: the culture of the workplace, the component tasks of a job, contact with co-workers, and the work environment. Finally a brainstorming exercise was used to generate some notional job titles for the individual. All team members were involved in this process in order to generate as many ideas as possible and to attempt to raise service workers expectations of the people they support.

Stage 2: Job development

Once notional job titles were arrived at, the task of job development could begin. McLoughlin et al. (1987) describe various job develop-ment techniques, but the Merseyside project tended to favour one particular method because of the need to develop highly individual-ized opportunities for severely disabled people.

Employers were approached on behalf of each disabled individual. The initial meeting was used to establish the needs of the employer, discuss the needs of the disabled person, and to describe the benefits of recruiting through our agency. Subsequent appointments were needed to visit the work site and focus attention on specific tasks and responsibilities which the individual could be employed to under-take. This was a particular area of expertise of the team social worker.

Many individuals started their working life with a job for two or three hours per week. This gave them the opportunity to build up their physical and mental stamina for work, and allowed them to make use of the 'therapeutic earnings' rule which allows a small amount of money to be earned without the reduction of State benefits.

Stage 3: Job training and support

A thorough analysis of the job was carried out by the job trainer in order to confirm the job match (McLoughlin, 1987). All job trainers used systematic instruction to teach work skills (Gold, 1980) and, where necessary, individualized adaptations were used to remove any physical barriers to the person doing the job. Adaptations were made to tools, equipment, the work environment, and the working method. The team occupational therapist had particular expertise in using adaptations to facilitate inclusion of disabled people. Some on-going support was provided by the disabled person's co-workers.

Stage 4: Evaluation

Regular reviews were seen as an essential part of the process. Because many of the disabled individuals did not communicate verbally, it was part of the job trainer's role to be aware of any behaviour that the individual used to communicate satisfaction or dissatisfaction with the service. Reviews also ensured that people could progress along a career path and move from unpaid work to a paid appointment. The team clinical psychologist took a lead in developing review procedures.

Conclusion

The success of this project has led to its expansion within Merseyside. It is also the subject of a research project being carried out by the University of Durham and Cleveland Psychology and Counselling. We hope that its success will lead to supported employment services nationally for multiply disabled people, and that this will both raise their expectations and provide them with new opportunities.

(I would like to acknowledge my co-workers on this project, Gillian Goodwin (social worker) and Jim William (top-grade clinical psychologist).)

References

Baumgart, D., Brown, L., Pumpian, I. et al. (1982) Principle of partial participation and individualized adaptation in educational programs for severely handicapped students. *Journal of the Association for Persons with Severe Handicaps*, **7 (2)**, 17–27

Brost, T. and Johnson, V. (1982) *Getting to Know You*, Wisconsin Coalition for Advocacy, Madison

Brown, L., Sharinga, B., York, J. et al. (1984) The direct pay waiver for severely intellectually handicapped workers. Unpublished manuscript, University of Wisconsin. Cited in *Getting Employed—Staying Employed*, (eds G. S. McLoughlin, J. B. Garner and M. Callahan) (1987), Paul H. Brookes, Baltimore

Gold, M. W. (1980) *Try Another Way: Training Manual*, Champaign, Research Press

National Development Team (1992) *Survey of Support Employment Services in England, Scotland and Wales*, Manchester

O'Brien, J. (1987) *A Framework For Accomplishment*, Responsive Systems Associates, Decatur

O'Brien, J. (1990) *Working On—a Survey of Emerging Issues in Supported Employment for People with Severe Disabilities*, Responsive Systems Associates, Georgia

Potts, M. and Fido, R. (1991) *A Fit Person to be Removed*: Personal Accounts of Life in a Mental Deficiency Institution, Northcote House, Plymouth

Ryan, J. and Thomas, F. (1987) *The Politics of Mental Handicap*, Free Association Books, London

These three accounts show health professionals beginning to work within the social model of disability, where disabled people are given a voice and greater control over their lives. Although the practices described are not beyond criticism (some people may think they do not go far enough), they show what can be done at the present time to improve services and enhance the quality of life of severely disabled people.

Index